Embodied Pleasure

A Solo Woman's Guide to Tantric Sexuality and Yoni Healing

Latasha Henrietta Hazra

ISBN: 978-1-7642608-6-2

Table of Contents

Chapter 1: Reclaiming Your Sacred Sensuality

You're reading this book for a reason. Maybe you picked it up because something inside you whispers that there's more to your sexuality than what you've experienced so far. Or perhaps you're tired of feeling disconnected from your body, from your pleasure, from that wild, sensual part of yourself that society taught you to hide. Could be you're curious about this whole "sacred sexuality" thing but don't know where to start.

Here's what I know: every woman carries within her an incredible capacity for pleasure, power, and spiritual connection through her sexuality. This isn't some new-age fantasy or wishful thinking. It's your birthright, and it's been systematically trained out of you since you were young.

What Sacred Sexuality Means for Modern Women

Sacred sexuality isn't about perfumed candles and pretending you're a goddess (unless that's your thing). At its core, it's about recognizing that your sexual energy is creative life force energy - the same power that grows babies, births ideas, and fuels your passion for living. When you treat this energy as sacred, you're simply acknowledging its true nature: powerful, transformative, and worthy of respect.

For modern women, this means something revolutionary. It means you get to define your own relationship with pleasure. You don't need anyone's permission to explore your body. You don't need to wait for the "right" partner to awaken your sensuality. And you definitely don't need to separate your spiritual life from your sexual life anymore.

Think about it. We live in a culture that simultaneously oversexualizes women's bodies while shaming women for actually enjoying those bodies. We're told to be sexy but not sexual. Desirable but not desiring. Available but not eager. No wonder so many of us feel confused, disconnected, or downright frustrated when it comes to our sexuality.

Sacred sexuality offers a different path. It says: Your pleasure matters. Your desires are valid. Your body is wise. And when you connect with your sexual energy consciously, you're not just having better orgasms (though that's certainly a nice bonus). You're tapping into a profound source of healing, creativity, and personal power.

Sarah, a 42-year-old teacher, came to understand this after years of unsatisfying relationships. "I always thought good sex meant making my partner happy," she told me. "I'd perform pleasure rather than feel it. When I started practicing sacred sexuality, everything changed. For the first time, I was present in my own body. I discovered I could have full-body orgasms just from breathing. I learned my yoni had been numb from years of disconnection, and as I healed that numbness, I healed other parts of my life too."

The beauty of sacred sexuality for modern women? It meets you exactly where you are. Single? Perfect. You can develop a profound relationship with your own body. In a partnership? Great. You can deepen your connection while maintaining your autonomy. Healing from trauma? These practices offer gentle, self-directed ways to reclaim your body. Postpartum? Menopausal? Dealing with illness? There's a practice for you.

Distinguishing Neo-Tantra from Traditional Practices

Now, let's address the elephant in the room. The practices in this book draw from tantric traditions that originated in India and Tibet over 5,000 years ago. But what you'll learn here isn't traditional Tantra with a capital T. That's a complex spiritual system involving years of study, specific initiations, and practices that go way beyond sexuality.

What we're exploring is often called neo-tantra - a Western adaptation that focuses primarily on the sexual and energetic practices while leaving behind many of the religious and cultural elements. And yes, we need to talk about cultural appropriation (Urban, 1999).

Traditional Tantra emerged within specific cultural contexts. In Hindu and Buddhist traditions, it encompasses elaborate rituals, deity worship, complex philosophical systems, and yes, some sexual practices - but those were just one small part of a much larger spiritual path. When Tantra came to the West in the 1960s and '70s, it got simplified, sexualized, and packaged for Western consumption.

This isn't necessarily bad, but it's important to be honest about what we're doing. We're taking tools and techniques that have proven helpful for connecting with sexual energy and adapting them for our modern context. We're not pretending to be Hindu or Buddhist practitioners. We're not claiming to teach "authentic" Tantra. We're acknowledging the roots while creating something new.

Think of it like yoga. Most Western yoga classes don't teach the full eight limbs of Patanjali's classical yoga system. They focus on the physical postures (asana) and maybe some breathing (pranayama). Similarly, neo-tantra focuses on specific techniques for working with sexual energy while leaving behind the broader religious context.

Here's what distinguishes neo-tantra from traditional practices:

Traditional Tantra:

- Requires initiation from a qualified guru
- Involves complex deity visualization
- Includes elaborate rituals and mantras
- Views sexual practices as one small part of a larger system
- Embedded in Hindu or Buddhist religious frameworks
- Often involves celibacy or highly controlled sexual practices
- Focuses on spiritual liberation as the primary goal

Neo-Tantra (What We're Practicing):

- Open to anyone who wants to learn
- Focuses on body awareness and energy work
- Adapts practices for modern lifestyles
- Centers sexual healing and pleasure
- Secular or spiritually inclusive
- Encourages conscious exploration of sexuality
- Aims for personal empowerment and healing

Understanding this distinction matters. When we practice neo-tantra with awareness of its origins, we can be respectful while still benefiting from these powerful techniques. We can acknowledge that we're part of a Western movement that's taken inspiration from Eastern traditions without claiming to represent those traditions.

Maria, a 35-year-old graphic designer, struggled with this at first. "I felt guilty, like I was stealing from another culture," she shared. "But then I realized - these practices were helping me heal from sexual trauma. I wasn't pretending to be something I'm not. I was using tools that worked, while respecting where they came from."

Your Journey Map Through This Book

So where are we going together? This book is structured as a journey, and like any good journey, it helps to have a map. You don't have to follow it perfectly - in fact, I encourage you to trust your instincts and explore what calls to you. But here's the general terrain we'll cover:

Part I: Foundations (Where You Are Now) We're starting with the basics because, honestly, most of us need to unlearn before we can learn. You'll discover how to work with your feminine energy (and no, that doesn't mean you have to be stereotypically "feminine"). You'll learn to create sacred space - both externally in your environment and internally in your mindset. And you'll master breathwork techniques that form the foundation of everything else.

Part II: Solo Sacred Practices This is where things get juicy. You'll learn to love yourself - literally. We'll explore yoni massage not as a quick route to orgasm but as a profound healing practice. You'll discover how your breasts connect to your heart and how that connection opens new pathways to pleasure. And yes, we'll talk about energy orgasms and full-body pleasure that doesn't depend on genital stimulation.

Why start with solo practices? Because sacred sexuality begins with your relationship with yourself. You can't share what you don't have. You can't receive what you don't believe you deserve. And you certainly can't communicate your needs if you don't know what they are.

Part III: Sacred Partnership Practices Once you've established a practice with yourself, you might choose to share these explorations with a partner. Notice I said "might" and "choose." This isn't required. But if you do have a partner (or partners), this section will help you navigate conscious communication, sacred touch, and mindful intimacy. You'll learn how to slow down, tune in, and create sexual experiences that nourish both of you.

5

Part IV: Integration and Transformation The final section helps you weave these practices into your daily life. We'll address the big stuff - healing sexual trauma, navigating different life stages, creating sustainable practice. Because sacred sexuality isn't just something you do in the bedroom. It's a way of living that honors your body, your energy, and your wholeness.

Throughout this journey, you'll meet women like yourself. Some of their stories might mirror your own. Others might surprise you. All of them remind us that there's no one "right" way to explore sacred sexuality. There's only your way.

You'll also find specific practices clearly marked. Some are daily practices you can do in five minutes. Others are longer rituals for when you have time and space. Many can be adapted to your needs. If you're a mom with young kids, your practice might look different than if you're single with lots of free time. That's perfect. This path honors your real life, not some fantasy version of it.

A Few Important Notes Before We Continue

First, this book assumes you're an adult woman making conscious choices about your body and sexuality. If you're dealing with active trauma, severe depression, or other mental health challenges, please work with a qualified therapist alongside these practices. Sacred sexuality can be profoundly healing, but it's not a replacement for professional help when you need it.

Second, you'll notice I use various terms for female anatomy. "Yoni" is a Sanskrit word meaning "sacred space" or "source." I'll use it interchangeably with vagina, vulva, and pussy - whatever feels right in the moment. You get to choose which words resonate for you. Language matters, and reclaiming how we name our bodies is part of reclaiming our power.

Third, while this book is written for women, it's inclusive of all women. If you have a yoni, this book is for you. Your sexual orientation doesn't matter. Your relationship status doesn't matter. Your age, size, ability, or background don't matter. Sacred sexuality is for every woman who wants to explore it.

Finally, take what serves you and leave the rest. You might love some practices and feel neutral about others. Perfect. You might need to adapt certain techniques for your body or situation. Please do. This isn't about following rules. It's about discovering what brings you alive.

The Invitation

Right now, in this moment, you're being invited into something profound. Not by me, but by your own deep wisdom. The part of you that picked up this book. The part that knows there's more to experience, more to feel, more to become.

This invitation doesn't require you to be different than you are. It doesn't need you to be more spiritual, more sexual, more anything. It simply asks you to be curious. To be willing. To consider that maybe - just maybe - your body holds wisdom you haven't accessed yet. Your pleasure contains medicine you haven't taken. Your sexuality offers a pathway to parts of yourself you haven't met.

You don't have to believe any of this yet. Skepticism is welcome here. So is fear, excitement, curiosity, and whatever else you're feeling. All of you is welcome on this journey.

What matters is that you're here. You're reading these words. You're considering the possibility that your relationship with your body and sexuality could be different. Could be more. Could be sacred.

And from where I'm sitting, that's already sacred. That's already brave. That's already the beginning of reclaiming what's always been yours.

So take a breath. Really, right now. Take a deep breath and let it out slowly. Feel your body in this moment. Notice where you're holding tension. Notice where you feel open. Notice without trying to change anything.

This is where we begin. Not with exotic techniques or esoteric knowledge. But with this simple act of presence. You, here, now, in your body, exactly as you are.

Welcome to your journey home.

Key Takeaways from This Chapter

- Sacred sexuality recognizes your sexual energy as creative life force, worthy of respect and conscious cultivation
- Modern sacred sexuality empowers women to define their own relationship with pleasure, independent of cultural shame or limitation
- Neo-tantra differs from traditional Tantra - we're adapting specific techniques while respecting their cultural origins
- This journey starts with solo practice because your relationship with yourself forms the foundation for everything else
- You're invited to take what serves you and adapt everything to your unique life circumstances
- Sacred sexuality isn't about becoming someone different - it's about coming home to who you already are

Chapter 2:Feminine Energy and Power

Let me guess - when you hear "feminine energy," part of you cringes a little. Maybe you picture flowing skirts, goddess circles, and women who speak in whispers about moon cycles. Or maybe you think it means being passive, receptive, and sweet all the time.

Here's the thing: feminine energy has nothing to do with how feminine you feel or act. You can rock a power suit and still be deeply connected to your feminine energy. You can be assertive, ambitious, and strong while fully embodying this power. Because feminine energy isn't about gender performance - it's about a quality of life force that everyone has access to, but that women are particularly wired to experience through our bodies.

The Science and Spirituality of Women's Sexuality

Your body is basically a biological marvel when it comes to sexual energy. And I'm not just saying that to make you feel good (though hopefully it does). Science backs this up in ways that would make your high school biology teacher blush.

Let's start with your clitoris. You probably learned it's that little button at the top of your vulva, right? Wrong. That's just the tip of the iceberg - literally. Your clitoris is actually a complex internal structure with over 8,000 nerve endings in the glans alone (Di Marino & Lepidi, 2014). It extends inside your body with two legs (crura) that are about 3-4 inches long, and two bulbs that surround your vaginal opening. When you get aroused, the whole structure becomes engorged with blood, creating sensation throughout your entire pelvic region.

But wait, there's more. Your vaginal canal is lined with nerve endings that respond to pressure, movement, and energy. Your G-spot (or G-zone, since it's not really a single spot) is an area of tissue on the front vaginal wall that swells when aroused. Some researchers now call it the female prostate because it can produce ejaculatory fluid (Komisaruk & Whipple, 2011).

Then there's your cervix - often ignored in conventional sex but considered the "heart of the yoni" in tantric traditions. Your cervix has three types of nerves: sympathetic (connecting to your heart and breath), parasympathetic (connecting to your digestion and grounding), and pelvic (connecting to your genitals). This means cervical stimulation can create full-body responses that feel emotional, spiritual, and physical all at once.

Why am I telling you all this anatomy? Because most of us grow up thinking we have one or two buttons down there, and if they don't work like they do in movies, something's wrong with us. But you're working with complex, interconnected systems designed for varied, nuanced experiences of pleasure.

Now here's where science meets spirituality. When you experience sexual arousal and orgasm, your brain releases a cocktail of chemicals:

- Oxytocin (the bonding hormone)
- Endorphins (natural pain killers)
- Dopamine (pleasure and reward)
- Serotonin (mood regulation)
- Prolactin (satisfaction and relaxation)

This chemical cascade doesn't just feel good - it literally changes your state of consciousness. Brain scans show that during orgasm, parts of your brain associated with behavioral control and fear basically go offline (Georgiadis et al., 2007). You enter an altered state similar to deep meditation or spiritual experience.

Traditional tantric texts described this thousands of years ago without the benefit of fMRI machines. They recognized that sexual energy, consciously cultivated, could produce mystical states. They mapped energy channels in the body that modern science is just beginning to understand through research on fascia, nerve networks, and bioelectric fields.

Jessica, a 38-year-old scientist, found this blend of science and spirituality transformative: "I needed to understand the 'why' before I could relax into the practice. Learning about my anatomy and neurology gave me permission to explore. Then when I had my first cervical orgasm, I understood what mystics meant by 'touching the divine.' It was like every cell in my body lit up at once."

Chakras and Energy Systems Specific to Women

Now let's talk about energy systems. In tantric traditions, chakras are energy centers that run along your spine. While everyone has these centers, women often experience them differently due to our cyclical nature and our capacity for creating life.

The traditional seven chakra system works like this:

1. **Root Chakra (Muladhara)** - Located at your perineum/pelvic floor
   - Governs: Safety, security, belonging
   - For women: Deeply connected to our sense of home in our bodies
2. **Sacral Chakra (Svadhisthana)** - Located below your navel
   - Governs: Sexuality, creativity, emotions
   - For women: The seat of our creative/sexual power, includes womb space
3. **Solar Plexus Chakra (Manipura)** - Located at your solar plexus

11

- o Governs: Personal power, will, confidence
- o For women: Often where we store beliefs about our worth
4. **Heart Chakra (Anahata)** - Located at your heart center
   - o Governs: Love, compassion, connection
   - o For women: Bridges sexual energy with emotional intimacy
5. **Throat Chakra (Vishuddha)** - Located at your throat
   - o Governs: Expression, truth, communication
   - o For women: Essential for expressing desires and boundaries
6. **Third Eye Chakra (Ajna)** - Located between your eyebrows
   - o Governs: Intuition, vision, wisdom
   - o For women: Heightened during menstruation and menopause
7. **Crown Chakra (Sahasrara)** - Located at the crown of your head
   - o Governs: Spiritual connection, unity consciousness
   - o For women: Opens naturally during childbirth and deep orgasmic states

But here's what many traditional systems miss: women have additional energy centers specific to our bodies. The breasts contain significant energy centers connected to both giving and receiving love. The womb space (whether or not you have a physical uterus) is a powerful creative center that exists energetically.

When working with your energy system, remember you're not trying to "fix" anything. You're simply bringing awareness to these centers and noticing what you find. Some might feel vibrant and open. Others might feel dense or closed. All of it is information, not judgment.

Anna, a massage therapist, describes her discovery: "I always felt disconnected from my solar plexus - that power center. Through breathwork and movement, I realized I'd been storing decades of 'good girl' programming there. As I breathed into that space and moved my hips, I literally felt old beliefs breaking up and moving out."

Monthly Cycles as Spiritual Practice

Okay, let's talk about something that might blow your mind: your menstrual cycle is basically a built-in spiritual practice. I know, I know. Most of us were taught to see our periods as inconvenient at best, shameful at worst. But what if I told you that your monthly cycle gives you access to different types of energy and wisdom throughout the month?

If you menstruate, your cycle mirrors the cycles of nature:

Menstrual Phase (Days 1-5ish) - Winter/New Moon Your energy turns inward. Your left and right brain hemispheres are most balanced during bleeding, giving you access to deep intuition (Pope, 2001). Many women report vivid dreams, psychic insights, and a need for solitude during this time. Instead of pushing through with caffeine and painkillers, what if you honored this as a time for rest and visioning?

Follicular Phase (Days 6-13ish) - Spring/Waxing Moon Energy starts rising. You feel more social, creative, optimistic. Your body is preparing for ovulation, and you might notice increased cervical fluid and sensitivity. This is a powerful time for starting new projects and practices. Your brain is particularly good at learning new things during this phase.

Ovulatory Phase (Days 14-16ish) - Summer/Full Moon Peak energy and magnetism. You're biologically primed to attract and connect. Your communication skills are enhanced, your skin glows, and your sexual energy is at its peak. Many women find this is when they have the easiest access to multiple orgasms and expanded pleasure states.

Luteal Phase (Days 17-28ish) - Autumn/Waning Moon
Energy begins turning inward again. Despite what PMS culture tells us, this can be a powerful time for discrimination and truth-telling. Your brain's right hemisphere becomes more active, enhancing intuition and creative problem-solving. Yes, you might feel more critical - but what if that criticism contains wisdom about what needs to change in your life?

For women who don't menstruate (due to menopause, hysterectomy, hormonal birth control, or other reasons), you can still work with cyclical energy by following the moon phases or seasons. Your body remembers rhythms even when the physical bleeding stops.

Rachel, 44, shared her experience: "I thought menopause meant losing my cyclical wisdom. But I started tracking the moon phases and noticed I still had energetic cycles. Now I plan my month around these subtle shifts. My 'inner winter' during the new moon is just as powerful as when I bled."

The key is tracking your own patterns. Use a journal or app to note:

- Energy levels
- Sexual desire
- Emotional states
- Creative impulses
- Dreams
- Physical sensations

After a few months, you'll see your unique patterns emerge. Maybe you're horniest right before your period, not during ovulation. Maybe your most creative time is during menstruation. There's no "right" pattern - only your pattern.

Working with Feminine and Masculine Energies

Here's something that might sound contradictory after a chapter on feminine energy: you also have masculine energy, and it's equally important. We all contain both energies, regardless of our gender identity. Think of them as different modes of being, not as gendered prescriptions.

Feminine Energy Qualities:

- Receptive and responsive
- Intuitive and feeling-based
- Cyclical and changing
- Being-focused
- Collaborative
- Process-oriented
- Surrendered

Masculine Energy Qualities:

- Active and initiating
- Logical and thinking-based
- Linear and consistent
- Doing-focused
- Competitive
- Goal-oriented
- Directed

In our culture, we've been trained to value masculine energy almost exclusively. We're rewarded for being productive, goal-oriented, and consistent. We're taught to override our bodies' signals and push through.

But here's what happens when we're always in masculine mode: we burn out. We lose touch with our intuition. We forget how to receive. We become uncomfortable with uncertainty and change.

Our sexuality becomes goal-oriented (must have orgasm!) rather than pleasure-oriented.

Sacred sexuality invites you to reclaim your feminine energy - not instead of your masculine energy, but in balance with it. You need both. Your masculine energy helps you create boundaries, make decisions, and take action. Your feminine energy helps you feel, flow, and receive.

Lisa, a CEO, learned this the hard way: "I was killing it in business but dying inside. I couldn't orgasm without my vibrator on the highest setting. I was so locked in masculine energy that I couldn't soften enough to receive pleasure. Learning to dance between both energies saved not just my sex life but my sanity."

The Power of Polarity

Whether you're solo or partnered, working with polarity - the dance between masculine and feminine energies - can amplify your experience. This isn't about gender roles. It's about energetic dynamics.

In solo practice, you can play with being both the giver (masculine) and receiver (feminine) of pleasure. Use one hand to actively stimulate while the other receives. Alternate between directing your breath and letting it flow naturally. Switch between focusing intently and surrendering to sensation.

With a partner, you can consciously play with these roles. One person holds more masculine energy (initiating, penetrating - with fingers, toys, or anatomy), while the other holds more feminine energy (receiving, responding, flowing). Then switch. Notice how different it feels to be in each role.

Same-sex couples often have more freedom here because they're not locked into anatomical assumptions about who should hold which energy. But regardless of your partner's gender, you can explore this dance.

The Dark Feminine

We need to talk about an aspect of feminine energy that's often ignored in "love and light" spiritual circles: the dark feminine. This isn't negative or bad. It's the part of feminine energy connected to destruction, transformation, and fierce boundaries.

Think of Kali in Hindu tradition - the goddess who destroys in order to create. Or the crone archetype who holds wisdom through witnessing death and rebirth. This energy knows how to say no, how to end what's not serving, how to compost the old to fertilize the new.

In your sexuality, the dark feminine might show up as:

- Fierce boundaries around your pleasure
- The ability to end relationships that don't serve you
- Rage that needs expression before softness can emerge
- The death of old sexual patterns
- Wild, primal expressions of pleasure

Many women fear this aspect because we've been taught to be nice, accommodating, and gentle. But the dark feminine is part of your wholeness. She's not cruel - she's precise. She's not destructive for destruction's sake - she clears space for what's real.

Monica discovered this during a yoni massage practice: "I was breathing into my cervix when suddenly rage erupted. Not at anyone specific, just old, old anger about all the ways my sexuality had been controlled. I roared and cried and shook. Afterwards, I felt empty in the best way - like I'd cleared space for something new."

Emotional Wisdom and Sexual Energy

Your emotions and sexual energy are intimately connected. This might seem obvious, but most of us are taught to separate them. We learn that "good sex" means leaving our emotions at the door. That we shouldn't cry during sex. That feeling sad or angry means we're not in the mood.

But your yoni doesn't lie. She holds emotional memory in her tissues. She contracts when she doesn't feel safe. She goes numb when there's unprocessed emotion. She can't fully open when your heart is closed.

This is actually brilliant design. Your sexual energy is so powerful that your body won't let it fully flow when there's emotional blocks. It's like a safety mechanism - deal with the feelings first, then we'll talk about pleasure.

Working with this connection means:

- Letting emotions move during self-pleasure or sex
- Understanding that numbness often covers emotion
- Recognizing that arousal can bring up unexpected feelings
- Knowing that emotional release can lead to deeper pleasure

Sandra, a therapist, shares: "I used to think I was broken because I'd cry after orgasm. Now I understand it as my body's way of releasing stored emotion. The orgasm opens the channel, and whatever needs to move, moves. Sometimes it's tears, sometimes laughter, sometimes sounds I didn't know I could make."

Reclaiming Your Sexual Power

So what does it mean to reclaim your feminine sexual power? It's not about becoming some idealized version of a "goddess." It's about coming home to what's already yours.

Your power lives in:

- Your ability to feel deeply
- Your capacity for multiple types of orgasms
- Your cyclical wisdom
- Your intuitive knowing
- Your creative/sexual life force
- Your emotional intelligence
- Your energetic sensitivity

But here's the radical truth: you don't have to earn this power. You don't have to be healed enough, spiritual enough, or sexy enough. This power is yours by birthright. It might be buried under layers of conditioning, trauma, or disconnection. But it's there, waiting.

The practices in this book are simply ways to remove the blocks. To clear the channel. To remember what your body has always known.

As you continue this journey, you might notice:

- Increased sensitivity to energy (your own and others')
- Clearer intuition about what you need
- Less tolerance for relationships that don't honor you
- More magnetism and presence
- Deeper capacity for pleasure
- Stronger sense of your own rhythm

These aren't signs that you're becoming someone new. They're signs that you're returning to who you've always been beneath the conditioning.

Your feminine energy isn't separate from your power - it IS your power. Not power over others, but power from within. The power to create, to transform, to feel, to know, to receive, to give from fullness rather than depletion.

This is what awaits as you continue this journey. Not perfection, but wholeness. Not constant bliss, but authentic aliveness. Not a fantasy of feminine energy, but the real, raw, revolutionary truth of who you are.

Key Takeaways from This Chapter

- Your sexual anatomy is far more complex and capable than most of us learned, with interconnected systems designed for varied pleasure
- Sexual arousal creates altered states of consciousness similar to meditation or spiritual experience
- Women have specific energy centers related to breasts and womb space beyond the traditional chakra system
- Your menstrual cycle (or energetic cycle) provides different types of power and wisdom throughout the month
- Balancing feminine and masculine energies enhances both solo and partnered experiences
- The dark feminine - connected to boundaries and transformation - is essential for wholeness
- Emotions and sexual energy are intimately connected; feeling deeply enhances pleasure
- Your feminine sexual power is your birthright, not something you need to earn

Chapter 3: Creating Sacred Space

You know that feeling when you walk into a room and immediately feel at ease? Or conversely, when you enter a space and your whole body tenses up? That's because spaces hold energy, and your body reads that energy faster than your mind can process it. Creating sacred space for your sensual practice isn't about fancy altars or expensive crystals (though if those call to you, great). It's about consciously crafting an environment - both external and internal - that tells your nervous system: you're safe here. You can open here. You can feel here.

Preparing Your Environment and Mindset

Let's start with a truth that might sting a little: most of us treat our sexuality as an afterthought. We squeeze it into the margins of our lives, between laundry and emails, in beds covered with unfolded clothes or while scrolling through our phones. Then we wonder why we feel disconnected from our pleasure.

Your environment matters because your body is always responding to its surroundings. When you're in a cluttered, chaotic space, part of your awareness stays vigilant. When you're in a beautiful, intentional space, your nervous system can relax into receptivity.

But here's what I'm not saying: I'm not saying you need a perfect temple room dedicated to sacred sexuality. Most of us are working with real-life constraints - kids, roommates, small apartments, busy schedules. Sacred space is about intention, not perfection.

Start with your bedroom. Look around right now. What does this space communicate about how you value rest, pleasure, and intimacy? If your bedroom doubles as your office, storage room, and laundry folding station, your body gets mixed signals. This is a workspace. No wait, it's a rest space. Actually, it's a passion space. Your nervous system stays confused.

Jennifer, a single mom of two, transformed her tiny bedroom with simple changes: "I couldn't afford a makeover, so I just cleared the clutter. I got a small basket for my kids' toys that inevitably ended up in my room. I hung a scarf over my work laptop at night. I put a salt lamp by my bed. These tiny shifts told my body: this is where I come to be a woman, not just a mom."

Here's your basic sacred space checklist:

Physical Space:

- Clear clutter (especially work-related items)
- Clean sheets and comfortable bedding
- Lighting you can adjust (candles, lamps, or dimmer switches)
- Temperature that feels good on bare skin
- Privacy (lock that works, curtains that close)
- Something beautiful to look at (art, flowers, fabric)
- Pleasant scent (incense, essential oils, or just fresh air)

Practical Additions:

- Towels within reach
- Water bottle nearby
- Tissues accessible
- Natural massage oil (coconut, almond, or specialized blends)
- Any toys or tools you enjoy, cleaned and ready
- Journal and pen for insights

Optional Enhancements:

- Altar with meaningful objects
- Crystals (rose quartz for heart opening, carnelian for sexuality)
- Images or statues that inspire you
- Soft music or nature sounds
- Essential oils for different moods

The key is making these preparations beforehand. Nothing kills the mood faster than realizing you need to hunt for massage oil or that your roommate might barge in. Set yourself up for success.

Setting Intentions and Boundaries

Now for the internal space - arguably more important than the external. You can have the most beautiful room in the world, but if your mind is racing through tomorrow's to-do list or rehashing an argument, you won't be present for pleasure.

Setting an intention is like giving your practice a North Star. It's not a goal (goals are masculine energy - achieve this outcome). An intention is feminine energy - a quality you want to cultivate or explore.

Examples of intentions:

- "I intend to listen deeply to my body"
- "I intend to explore without judgment"
- "I intend to stay present with whatever arises"
- "I intend to soften into sensation"
- "I intend to celebrate my body exactly as it is"
- "I intend to release old patterns with compassion"

Notice these aren't: "I intend to have five orgasms" or "I intend to squirt." Those are goals. They create pressure. Intentions create space.

Maria learned this distinction through experience: "I used to start every session with goals - work on my G-spot, practice energy orgasms, whatever I'd read about. I was basically giving myself a sexual homework assignment. When I switched to intentions like 'I intend to be curious,' everything opened up. Ironically, that's when I started having the experiences I'd been chasing."

Boundaries are the container that holds your practice. Without them, your energy leaks out in a thousand directions. Boundaries aren't walls - they're more like the banks of a river that allow the water to flow with power.

Time boundaries:

- Decide how long your practice will be
- Turn off all devices or put them in another room
- Let household members know you need privacy
- Give yourself buffer time before and after

Energy boundaries:

- This practice is for you (not to please a future partner)
- You're not trying to prove anything
- You can stop anytime you want
- You don't have to push through discomfort

Mental boundaries:

- Critical thoughts are noted but not indulged
- Comparisons to others are acknowledged and released
- Performance pressure is recognized and set aside
- Past experiences don't dictate present exploration

Creating boundaries might feel selfish at first. Good. We need more women being "selfish" about their pleasure and well-being. The world won't fall apart if you take an hour for yourself. In fact, it might run better when you're resourced and connected to your power.

Self-Care as Spiritual Practice

Here's where we need to reclaim the concept of self-care from the commodified, commercialized version sold to us. Real self-care isn't about expensive face masks or spa days (though those can be lovely). It's about treating yourself as sacred. And that starts with the basics.

When was the last time you really inhabited your body during everyday care? Most of us shower on autopilot, thinking about everything except the warm water on our skin. We moisturize while checking emails. We eat while working. No wonder we feel disconnected.

Sacred self-care means bringing presence to these ordinary moments. It means treating your body as the temple it is - not in some ethereal, disconnected way, but in a grounded, practical way.

Try this: Next time you shower, arrive fully. Feel the temperature of the water. Notice how it hits different parts of your body. When you soap up, touch yourself like you would touch a lover - with attention, appreciation, maybe even arousal. When you dry off, pay attention to the texture of the towel, the awakening of your skin.

This isn't about making everything sexual. It's about making everything sensual - connected to your senses, your aliveness, your presence in this body.

Sophie discovered this after years of punishing exercise routines: "I used to work out to punish my body into submission. Now I dance to celebrate what my body can do. I moisturize like I'm giving myself a massage. I eat foods that make me feel vibrant, not virtuous. This shift in how I care for myself daily changed everything about my sexuality."

Creating Ritual vs. Routine

There's a difference between routine and ritual. Routine is autopilot - the things you do without thinking. Ritual is conscious, intentional, meaningful. It marks a transition from ordinary to sacred time.

You don't need elaborate rituals. Simple is often better. The point is to signal to your body-mind that you're entering sacred space.

A basic opening ritual might include:

1. **Cleansing** - Wash your hands and face, or take a shower
2. **Transition** - Change clothes or wrap yourself in something special
3. **Space clearing** - Light incense, ring a bell, or simply open windows
4. **Centering** - Sit quietly and take five deep breaths
5. **Intention setting** - Speak or write your intention
6. **Opening** - Place hands on heart and yoni, acknowledging your body

A closing ritual is equally important:

1. **Gratitude** - Thank your body for what it shared
2. **Integration** - Journal insights or simply rest
3. **Grounding** - Eat something, drink water, or touch the earth
4. **Transition** - Change clothes or wash face/hands

5. **Closing** - Blow out candles, close sacred space

The magic isn't in the specific actions. It's in the consciousness you bring. It's in telling your system: what happens here matters. This time is sacred. You are worth this attention.

Working with Resistance

Let's be honest - as you start creating sacred space and time for your practice, resistance will show up. Count on it. Your mind will offer a greatest hits compilation of why this is silly, selfish, or unnecessary.

Common forms of resistance:

- "I don't have time for this"
- "This feels too weird/woo-woo"
- "I should be doing something productive"
- "My space isn't nice enough"
- "I'm too tired/stressed/busy"
- "This is selfish when others need me"

Resistance is actually a good sign. It means you're approaching something that matters, something that could create real change. Your ego likes the status quo, even when the status quo includes numbness, disconnection, or dissatisfaction.

Instead of fighting resistance, get curious about it. What's underneath? Often it's fear:

- Fear of feeling too much
- Fear of discovering something painful
- Fear of wanting more than you have
- Fear of your own power
- Fear of change

Karen's resistance showed up as perpetual busyness: "I'd plan sacred time, then suddenly remember urgent emails or decide the bathroom needed cleaning. I realized I was terrified of being alone with my body without an agenda. What if I felt nothing? What if I felt everything? It took three weeks of showing up despite the resistance before my system trusted this new rhythm."

Energy Hygiene

Just like you shower to clean your physical body, you need practices to clean your energy body. This becomes especially important as you open to more sensation and sensitivity through sacred sexuality practices.

Everything you encounter leaves an energetic residue. The argument with your partner, the stressful meeting, the disturbing news story - all of it sticks to your energy field. If you don't clear it, you're carrying all that static into your sacred practice.

Simple energy clearing practices:

Salt Bath: Add 1-2 cups of sea salt or Epsom salt to a warm bath. Soak for 20 minutes, imagining the salt drawing out stagnant energy. This literally changes the electrical charge around your body.

Smoke Clearing: Burn sage, palo santo, or incense. Wave the smoke around your body, paying special attention to your heart and pelvic area. Indigenous cultures have used smoke clearing for thousands of years because it works.

Sound Clearing: Use a singing bowl, bells, or even your own voice. Sound breaks up stuck energy. Humming or toning while focusing on different parts of your body can shift your entire state.

Breath Clearing: Take sharp exhales through your mouth while shaking your body. This moves stagnant energy and resets your nervous system. Do this for 30-60 seconds, then stand still and notice the tingling aliveness.

Nature Clearing: Stand barefoot on earth, swim in natural water, or sit with your back against a tree. Nature literally grounds excess energy and recharges your system.

Creating Sacred Space in Challenging Circumstances

Real talk: sometimes life doesn't allow for perfect sacred space. You might be:

- Sharing space with kids who don't sleep
- Living with roommates and thin walls
- Dealing with a hostile or unsupportive partner
- Traveling or in temporary housing
- Managing illness or disability

Sacred space is ultimately an internal experience. Yes, external support helps. But women throughout history have found ways to connect with their sacred sexuality in convents, crowded homes, even prisons.

If you can't control your external space:

- Create sacred time in the shower or bath
- Use visualization to create internal temple space
- Practice while others are out of the house
- Find spots in nature for practice
- Use breathwork and subtle movement anywhere
- Claim even five minutes as sacred

Amanda, living in a studio apartment with her partner working from home during pandemic: "I created sacred space in my morning shower. Those 15 minutes became my temple. I'd set an intention, do breast massage, practice presence. It wasn't ideal, but it kept me connected to myself when everything else felt chaotic."

The Sacred in the Ordinary

Here's the ultimate secret about sacred space: everywhere is sacred when you bring sacred attention. The designation of certain spaces or times as "sacred" is really just practice for living all of life as sacred.

As you develop your practice, you might notice:

- Washing dishes becomes a sensual experience
- Walking becomes a moving meditation
- Eating becomes communion with life
- Breathing becomes prayer

This isn't about being serious or "spiritual" all the time. It's about being alive all the time. It's about not compartmentalizing your sensuality, your pleasure, your aliveness into one hour a week.

The women who thrive in sacred sexuality aren't the ones with perfect altars. They're the ones who find the sacred in folding laundry, who breathe into their bellies while stopped at red lights, who touch their own skin with reverence while applying sunscreen.

They understand that sacred space starts with the decision to treat yourself as sacred. Everything else flows from there.

Building Your Sacred Space Practice

Start where you are. Tonight, before bed, try this:

1. Clear one surface in your bedroom - nightstand, dresser top, doesn't matter

2. Place one beautiful thing on it - a flower, a candle, a photo that makes you smile
3. Sit on your bed and take five conscious breaths
4. Place one hand on your heart, one on your belly
5. Say (out loud or silently): "This is sacred space. I am sacred. My pleasure matters."

That's it. You've begun.

From this seed, your practice can grow. Maybe tomorrow you add a second beautiful thing. Maybe next week you clear a whole corner. Maybe next month you claim an hour of undisturbed time.

Or maybe you just keep it simple. Five breaths. Two hands on your body. One moment of recognition: this is sacred.

Because it is. You are. And the sooner you start living like you believe it, the sooner everything changes.

Key Takeaways from This Chapter

- Your environment directly impacts your nervous system's ability to relax into pleasure and presence
- Sacred space requires intention more than perfection - small changes can create big shifts
- Setting intentions (not goals) and boundaries creates an energetic container for your practice
- Real self-care means bringing sacred attention to ordinary body care
- Ritual marks the transition from ordinary to sacred time through conscious actions
- Resistance to creating sacred space often masks fear of feeling, changing, or claiming power
- Energy hygiene is as important as physical hygiene when working with expanded sensitivity

- Sacred space is ultimately an internal experience you can cultivate anywhere

Chapter 4: Breathwork and Body Awareness

Your breath is the bridge between your conscious mind and your unconscious body. Right now, you're probably breathing just enough to stay alive - shallow sips of air that keep you functional but not much more. What if I told you that learning to breathe differently could unlock pleasure you didn't know existed? That your breath could be the key to full-body orgasms, emotional release, and states of consciousness usually reserved for deep meditation?

Most of us breathe backwards. Watch a baby breathe - their whole belly moves, soft and easy. Then watch most adults - chest breathing, shoulders rising, belly held tight. We learned to suck in our stomachs and puff out our chests. We learned that taking up space, even with our breath, wasn't ladylike. And in doing so, we cut ourselves off from our power source.

Foundational Breathing Techniques

Before we dive into specific techniques, let's assess where you're starting. Place one hand on your chest, one on your belly. Take a normal breath. Which hand moves more? If it's the chest hand, you're not alone. But you're also not breathing optimally for pleasure, relaxation, or energy flow.

Belly Breathing (Natural Breathing)

This is where everything starts. It's so simple that your mind might reject it as "not enough." Trust me, master this first.

1. Lie down or sit comfortably with spine straight
2. Place both hands on your belly

3. Exhale completely through your mouth
4. Close your mouth and inhale slowly through your nose
5. Let your belly expand like a balloon filling
6. Exhale through your nose, belly falling naturally
7. Continue for 5-10 breaths

The trick? Your chest shouldn't move much. This might feel weird at first. You might feel like you're not getting enough air. That's just your system adjusting to actually getting more oxygen than usual.

Practice this throughout your day. While driving. While cooking. While watching TV. The more natural belly breathing becomes, the more your whole system shifts into receptivity.

Connected Breathing (Circular Breathing)

This technique, used in various forms from rebirthing to holotropic breathwork, creates an altered state within minutes. It's powerful, so start slowly.

1. Lie down in your sacred space
2. Begin breathing in and out through your mouth
3. Make the breath continuous - no pause between inhale and exhale
4. Keep it gentle and rhythmic, like waves
5. If you feel tingling or lightheadedness, slow down
6. Continue for 5-10 minutes to start

What you might experience:

- Tingling in hands, feet, or face (totally normal)
- Emotional waves (let them move)
- Energy moving through your body
- Altered perception
- Spontaneous movement or sound

Lucy, a yoga teacher, describes her first experience: "I thought I knew breathwork. Then I tried connected breathing. Within minutes, I felt electricity running through my body. My yoni started pulsing without any touch. I cried, laughed, and had what I can only describe as an energy orgasm. All from breathing!"

Fire Breath (Bellows Breath)

This activating breath builds energy quickly. Use it when you feel sluggish or disconnected from your body.

1. Sit up straight, hands on belly
2. Take a deep breath in
3. Exhale sharply through your nose, pulling belly in
4. Let the inhale happen naturally as belly releases
5. Repeat rapidly - the exhale is active, inhale passive
6. Start with 20 breaths, work up to 50-100
7. After final exhale, inhale deeply and hold for 10 seconds
8. Release and breathe normally

Warning: This can make you dizzy. Don't do it standing up at first. Also avoid if you're pregnant, menstruating heavily, or have high blood pressure.

Breath of Arousal (Bliss Breath)

This specifically moves sexual energy through your body. It's like plugging yourself into an electrical socket.

1. Inhale through your nose, imagining breath entering your yoni
2. Pull the breath up your spine to the crown of your head
3. Hold for 3-5 seconds at the top
4. Exhale through your mouth with a soft "ahhhh" sound
5. Let the energy cascade down your front body
6. Repeat 10-20 times

Add pelvic floor engagement:

- On inhale: gently squeeze your pelvic floor muscles
- On hold: maintain gentle squeeze
- On exhale: completely release and soften

This breath alone can bring you to the edge of orgasm. Combined with touch, it's explosive.

Body Scanning and Tension Release

Now let's talk about your body awareness. Most of us live from the neck up, occasionally visiting our bodies for sex or exercise. But your body is constantly communicating through sensation. Learning its language changes everything.

The Basic Body Scan

Do this daily, preferably before any sacred sexuality practice:

1. Lie down comfortably, eyes closed
2. Start at the crown of your head
3. Slowly move your attention down your body
4. Notice without judging: tight, relaxed, numb, tingly, warm, cool
5. Spend extra time at: jaw, shoulders, heart, belly, pelvis, yoni
6. Don't try to change anything, just notice
7. Complete scan to your toes
8. Return to any areas calling for attention

What you're building is called interoception - awareness of internal sensation. Studies show that people with higher interoception have better sex, stronger emotional regulation, and greater overall well-being (Mehling et al., 2018).

Progressive Tension Release

Sometimes you need to tense to release. This technique helps you identify and let go of holding patterns.

1. Start with your feet
2. Tense all muscles in feet for 5 seconds
3. Release suddenly and completely
4. Notice the contrast for 10 seconds
5. Move up: calves, thighs, glutes, belly, chest, arms, shoulders, neck, face
6. Finally, tense your whole body at once
7. Release and melt into the surface beneath you
8. Rest in total relaxation for 5 minutes

Pay special attention to:

- Jaw (where we hold control)
- Shoulders (where we carry the world)
- Belly (where we store fear)
- Pelvic floor (where we grip against feeling)

Sarah discovered chronic pelvic tension this way: "I had no idea I was constantly clenching my pelvic floor. It was like I'd been wearing a corset inside my vagina for 30 years. When I learned to release, not only did sex stop hurting, but I started having vaginal orgasms for the first time."

Awakening Dormant Sensation

Here's a truth that might hurt: many women are numb in their erogenous zones. Not physically damaged, but energetically and neurologically disconnected. Years of rushing, forcing, overriding, or checking out during sex creates a kind of amnesia in our tissues.

The good news? Sensation can be reawakened. Your body wants to feel. It just needs safe, patient attention.

Mapping Your Sensation

Get curious about your current sensation map:

1. In sacred space, undress and lie down
2. Using clean hands and oil if desired
3. Touch different parts of your body with same pressure
4. Rate sensation on scale of 1-10 (1=numb, 10=extremely sensitive)
5. Map areas: breasts, nipples, inner arms, neck, belly, inner thighs, labia, clitoris, vaginal entrance, internal walls
6. No judgment - just data gathering

Common patterns:

- High sensation at clitoris, numbness internally
- Numb nipples but sensitive breasts
- More sensation on one side than the other
- Areas of hypersensitivity next to numb spots

Breast Awakening Practice

Your breasts are directly connected to your heart and yoni through nerve pathways and energy channels. Awakening breast sensation opens your whole system.

1. Cup your breasts gently
2. Breathe into your hands
3. Begin slow circles around the outside
4. Spiral inward toward nipples
5. Vary pressure: feather light to firm
6. Try different touches: tapping, squeezing, holding
7. Breathe arousal breath while touching
8. Continue for 10-15 minutes
9. Rest hands on breasts and notice

Don't chase arousal. Court sensation. There's a difference.

Yoni Awakening Practice

This is not masturbation as you know it. This is conscious touch for awakening.

1. Start with external massage: mons, outer labia
2. Use plenty of oil
3. Touch like you're touching sacred ground
4. Breathe into your touch
5. Notice without agenda: temperature, texture, sensation
6. Gently include inner labia, clitoris
7. If comfortable, include vaginal entrance
8. No goal except presence and breath
9. If arousal comes, breathe it through your body
10. End by cupping your whole yoni

Michelle's experience: "I'd been numbing out during sex for years. This practice was revolutionary. At first, I felt nothing except sadness about feeling nothing. I kept breathing, kept touching with presence. After a few weeks, sensation started returning. It was like color coming back to a black and white world."

Integration of Breath and Touch

Here's where magic happens - combining conscious breathing with awakened touch. Your breath directs energy. Your touch grounds it. Together, they create a circuit of pleasure that doesn't depend on friction or fantasy.

Basic Integration Practice:

1. Begin with 5 minutes of connected breathing
2. Continue breathing while beginning breast massage
3. Sync touch with breath: firmer on exhale, lighter on inhale
4. Move to yoni when ready

5. Breathe into your touch - literally imagine breath entering where you touch
6. If approaching orgasm, slow down and breathe deeper
7. Spread sensation with breath: inhale up spine, exhale down front
8. Continue as long as feels good
9. End with hands on heart and yoni, breathing gratitude

The Microcosmic Orbit

This Taoist practice circulates sexual energy through your whole system instead of letting it dissipate.

1. As arousal builds, inhale energy up your spine
2. Visualize it moving from yoni to sacrum to heart to crown
3. At crown, touch tongue to roof of mouth
4. Exhale down front channel: third eye to throat to heart to belly to yoni
5. Continue circulating: up back, down front
6. This prevents energy from getting "stuck" in genitals
7. Creates full-body pleasure waves

Working with Numbness and Hypersensitivity

Both numbness and hypersensitivity are forms of protection. Your body learned to dial down or amp up sensation for good reasons. Respect these patterns while gently inviting change.

For Numbness:

- Start with non-sexual body parts
- Use varied stimulation: temperature, texture, pressure
- Breathe into the numb area
- Make sound - humming or toning can wake up tissue
- Be patient - sensation returns slowly
- Consider emotional components

For Hypersensitivity:

- Begin with very light, indirect touch
- Breathe out on contact (releases bracing)
- Use flat palm vs. pointed fingers
- Work around the sensitive area first
- Short sessions with integration time
- Build tolerance gradually

Breath as Anchor

In all practices, breath is your anchor. When emotions arise, breathe. When sensation overwhelms, breathe. When you disconnect, breathe. When you want to rush, breathe.

Your breath tells your nervous system:

- Deep, slow breath = you're safe
- Held breath = danger, freeze
- Shallow breath = anxiety, vigilance
- Rhythmic breath = all is well

This is why conscious breathing during sexual practice (solo or partnered) changes everything. You're literally rewiring your nervous system to associate pleasure with safety.

Daily Breath Practices

To embody these teachings, weave breath awareness through your day:

Morning: 5 minutes belly breathing before getting up
Commute: Connected breathing at red lights **Work:** Fire breath between meetings for energy **Evening:** Body scan while cooking dinner **Bedtime:** Arousal breath to stay connected to eros

Creating Your Practice

Start simple. Choose one breathing technique and one awareness practice. Do them daily for a week before adding more. Your practice might look like:

Week 1: Belly breathing + basic body scan Week 2: Add connected breathing Week 3: Add breast awakening Week 4: Integrate breath with touch

Or create your own progression. The key is consistency over intensity. Five minutes daily transforms more than an hour once a week.

Remember: You're not trying to become a breathwork expert. You're learning to inhabit your body fully. To feel what's actually there. To move energy consciously. To wake up from the trance of disconnection.

Your breath has been waiting your whole life for you to discover its power. Your body has been holding sensation in trust until you were ready to feel. That time is now.

One breath at a time, you're coming home.

Key Takeaways from This Chapter

- Proper breathing starts with belly breathing - chest breathing limits both oxygen and energy flow
- Connected/circular breathing creates altered states and moves emotional and energetic blocks
- Different breath techniques serve different purposes: fire breath energizes, arousal breath moves sexual energy
- Body scanning builds interoception - your ability to feel internal sensation

- Many women experience numbness from disconnection, which can be reawakened through patient, conscious touch
- Combining breath with touch creates an energy circuit that amplifies pleasure
- The microcosmic orbit prevents sexual energy from getting "stuck" in genitals
- Consistency matters more than perfection - daily short practices transform more than sporadic long one

Chapter 5: The Art of Self-Love

Let's start with the elephant in the room: masturbation. Even the word might make you cringe a little. It sounds clinical, mechanical, vaguely shameful. Like something teenage boys do under covers, not something sacred or spiritual. We need better language for what we're really talking about here - making love to yourself, self-pleasure practice, solo cultivation. Because what you're about to learn has nothing to do with quickly rubbing one out before bed.

This is about revolutionizing your relationship with your own body. It's about becoming your own best lover. It's about discovering that you are both the seeker and the sought, the lover and the beloved. And that changes everything.

Reframing Masturbation as Spiritual Practice

Here's what nobody told you: every major spiritual tradition that included sexual practices recognized solo cultivation as essential. Not as a poor substitute for partnered sex, but as a powerful practice in its own right. The Taoists called it "solo cultivation." Tantrics called it "self-worship." They understood something we've forgotten - your sexual energy is your creative life force, and learning to cultivate it consciously is a spiritual act.

But somewhere along the way, we turned self-pleasure into something shameful. Something you do when you can't get the "real thing." Something quick and goal-oriented. Something to hide.

Think about the messages you received:

- Don't touch yourself there
- Nice girls don't do that
- It'll make you loose/damaged/unable to enjoy "real" sex
- It's selfish/sinful/wrong
- Only desperate people need to do that

No wonder most women either don't self-pleasure at all (studies suggest 20-40% of women rarely or never masturbate) or do it with a hefty side of shame (Kaestle & Allen, 2011). We've been robbed of one of our most powerful tools for self-knowledge, healing, and empowerment.

Here's what self-pleasure as spiritual practice actually offers:

- Complete sovereignty over your own body
- Understanding of your unique arousal patterns
- Healing from sexual trauma or negative conditioning
- Increased capacity for pleasure
- Stronger orgasms and new types of orgasmic experience
- Better communication with partners about your needs
- Direct access to creative/spiritual energy
- Deep self-love and acceptance

Rebecca, a 45-year-old therapist, shares: "I'd been married 20 years and never had an orgasm. I blamed my husband, my body, my hormones. When I finally started a self-pleasure practice, I realized I'd never taken responsibility for my own pleasure. Within a month, I was having multiple orgasms - alone and with my partner. But more importantly, I felt like I'd come home to myself."

Mirror Work and Body Acceptance

Before we get to touch, we need to talk about seeing. When was the last time you really looked at your vulva? Not a quick glance while inserting a tampon, but really looked? With curiosity, appreciation, maybe even awe?

Most women have never truly seen their own yonis. We can describe our faces in detail but not the gateway to life itself. This disconnection from our own anatomy keeps us dependent on others' opinions about our bodies.

Basic Mirror Practice:

1. Get a hand mirror and good lighting
2. Find comfortable position - lying down with knees bent, squatting, or sitting
3. Just look for 5 minutes without judgment
4. Notice colors, textures, shapes
5. Watch how everything changes as you breathe
6. Touch gently and watch the response
7. Say one appreciative thing out loud

Common reactions:

- "It's weird/ugly/not like porn"
- Fascination with the complexity
- Emotional waves - sadness, anger, joy
- Surprise at how much it changes
- Recognition of beauty

Your vulva is as unique as your face. The idea that there's a "normal" way to look is marketing BS designed to sell you labiaplasty and shame. Every vulva is perfect in its uniqueness.

Full Body Mirror Work:

This expands beyond genitals to your whole self:

1. Stand naked before a full-length mirror
2. Start with 30 seconds if that's all you can handle
3. Breathe and soften your gaze
4. Notice where your mind goes critical
5. For every criticism, find something to appreciate

6. Touch parts of your body while watching
7. Practice regularly until you can stand in appreciation

Anna's breakthrough: "I avoided mirrors for years. When I finally did this practice, I sobbed. I saw my mother's body, my grandmother's body. I saw the story of my life written in stretch marks and scars. Instead of hate, I felt tenderness. That shifted everything about how I touched myself."

Creating Self-Pleasure Rituals

Now we transform masturbation from quick release to sacred ritual. This doesn't mean it always has to be elaborate - sometimes you need quick connection. But having a full ritual practice changes your baseline relationship with self-pleasure.

Preparation Ritual:

1. **Set sacred space** - Clean room, fresh sheets, candles, music
2. **Cleanse** - Shower or bath with intention
3. **Adorn** - Oil your body, wear something beautiful (or nothing)
4. **Arrive** - Sit quietly, hands on heart and yoni
5. **Intention** - Speak your purpose for this practice
6. **Gratitude** - Thank your body for its wisdom

The Practice Itself:

Forget everything you think you know about masturbation. No racing to orgasm. No favorite fantasy on repeat. No vibrator on highest setting until you go numb. This is about presence, exploration, and letting your body lead.

Starting Slow:

- Begin with non-genital touch

47

- Massage your feet, legs, belly
- Include your whole body
- Dance, stretch, move
- Let arousal build naturally

Breast and Heart Connection:

- Spend 10-15 minutes on breast massage
- Connect heart and yoni energetically
- Many women need this to fully open

Approaching Your Yoni:

- Circle around before going direct
- Inner thighs, mons, outer labia
- Tease yourself awake
- Use lots of natural oil

Conscious Touch:

- Vary pressure: feather light to firm
- Vary speed: slow to quick
- Vary pattern: circles, strokes, tapping
- Include everything: clitoris, labia, entrance, internally
- Breathe into your touch

Edge Practice:

- Build arousal to 8/10
- Back off to 5/10
- Build again
- Creates stronger, fuller orgasms
- Teaches you your arousal arc

Integration:

- If you orgasm, breathe it through your whole body

- If you don't, celebrate the pleasure you felt
- Rest with hands on body
- Journal insights

Closing Ritual:

- Thank your body
- Ground with food/water
- Gentle movement
- Return to daily life slowly

Working with Fantasy and Presence

Here's a controversial truth: most women need fantasy to orgasm because they've never learned to be present with sensation. Fantasy isn't bad, but dependence on it disconnects you from your body's wisdom.

Try this experiment:

- Week 1: Notice your go-to fantasies without judgment
- Week 2: Alternate between fantasy and sensation focus
- Week 3: Practice one session purely sensation-focused
- Week 4: Choose consciously when to use fantasy

When focusing on sensation:

- Describe what you feel: "warm, tingly, pulsing"
- Breathe into the sensation
- Make sounds that express the feeling
- Move in ways that increase pleasure
- Stay curious about what wants to happen

Lisa discovered: "I realized I always fantasized about being desired because I didn't desire myself. When I started focusing on sensation, I had to confront that numbness. But as I stayed present, I found sensation I'd been overriding with mental

49

movies. Now I can choose - sometimes fantasy enhances, sometimes presence is enough."

Tools and Toys as Sacred Allies

Let's talk about vibrators and toys. They're not cheating. They're not replacing human touch. Used consciously, they're allies in your pleasure journey.

Choosing Consciously:

- Quality over quantity
- Body-safe materials only (silicone, glass, steel)
- Different tools for different practices
- Clean and charge as part of ritual

Types and Uses:

External vibrators:

- Great for awakening sensation
- Use on lowest setting first
- Move around whole vulva
- Try through fabric first

Dildos/Internal toys:

- For exploring internal sensation
- Different sizes for different practices
- Can help with de-armoring
- Useful for G-spot/cervical exploration

Crystal/Stone wands:

- For energy work
- Stay present - they don't vibrate
- Can help with emotional release

- Beautiful ritual objects

Natural options:

- Your beautiful fingers
- Organic coconut oil
- Warm water in bath
- Silk fabric
- Your own breath and sound

Remember: Tools are supplements, not replacements. If you can only orgasm with a vibrator on high, you've trained your nerves to need intense stimulation. Practice backing off, using lower settings, combining with breath and presence.

Cycles and Rhythms in Practice

Your self-pleasure practice will naturally ebb and flow with your cycles. Honor this instead of forcing consistency.

Menstrual Cycle Awareness:

During bleeding: Often deeply internal, may want no touch or very gentle external touch. Some women experience heightened sensation.

Pre-ovulation: Energy building, playful exploration, trying new things

Ovulation: Peak arousal for many, easiest orgasms, most open to penetration

Pre-menstruum: May feel more emotional, need slower approach, deeper internal work

Track your patterns. You might discover:

- Different types of touch feel good at different times
- Orgasms change quality throughout your cycle
- Certain practices work better in certain phases
- Your fantasies/desires shift cyclically

Life Seasons:

Your practice also shifts with life seasons:

- **Postpartum:** Gentle reconnection, lots of oil, patience
- **Perimenopause:** May need more time, different stimulation
- **Post-menopause:** Often a sexual renaissance with right approach
- **Times of stress:** Shorter practices, focus on regulation
- **Times of expansion:** Longer practices, new exploration

Healing Through Self-Pleasure

This practice heals more than sexual issues. Women report healing:

- Body shame and negative self-image
- Inability to receive (in all areas)
- Boundary issues
- Creative blocks
- Relationship patterns
- Trust issues
- Power dynamics

How? Because sexual energy is life force energy. When you heal your relationship with it, you heal your relationship with life itself.

Maria's story: "I started self-pleasure practice to fix my 'broken' orgasms. What I got was so much more. I found rage I'd been storing in my pelvis. Grief about all the years of disconnection.

Joy I didn't know existed. As I made love to myself, I learned to love myself. My whole life reorganized around that new foundation."

Common Challenges and Solutions

"I don't have time" Start with 5 minutes. Touch yourself with presence while moisturizing. Make breast massage part of your shower. Quality over quantity.

"I feel nothing/numb" Normal if you've been disconnected. Keep showing up with patience. Try temperature play (ice/warmth). Focus on areas with more sensation first. Consider emotional components.

"I get bored" You're probably goal-focused. Let go of orgasm as objective. Explore like you're mapping new territory. Try new positions, touches, rhythms.

"I feel guilty/ashamed" Notice the voices - whose are they? Not yours. Write down the shame stories and burn them. Start very simple - just holding your vulva with love.

"My mind won't stop racing" Use breath as anchor. Count breaths. Describe sensations out loud. Put on music that grounds you. This is mindfulness practice.

"I always cry" Beautiful! Your yoni holds emotion. Let it move. Have tissues ready. Know that tears often precede opening to greater pleasure.

Creating Your Personal Practice

Your practice will be unique. Here's a template to customize:

Daily (5 minutes):

- Morning breast massage in shower
- OR evening vulva holding before sleep
- OR conscious breathing touching heart/yoni

Weekly (30-60 minutes):

- Full ritual practice
- Include whole body
- Explore edge or new technique

Monthly (90+ minutes):

- Extended practice
- Try something new
- Include integration time
- Journal insights

Quarterly:

- Assess what's working/not working
- Adjust practice to life changes
- Celebrate progress
- Set new intentions

The Ripple Effect

Here's what women report after establishing consistent self-pleasure practice:

- Better orgasms (alone and partnered)
- Clearer boundaries in all areas
- Increased creativity and productivity
- Better body image
- Improved partner communication
- Stronger sense of self
- Increased magnetism
- Better health (immune, hormonal)

- Spiritual opening
- Life purpose clarity

This isn't magic. It's what happens when you stop abandoning yourself. When you stop waiting for someone else to unlock your pleasure. When you take radical responsibility for your own aliveness.

Integration Into Life

Self-pleasure practice doesn't exist in vacuum. It weaves into your whole life:

- Touch yourself with love throughout the day
- Breathe into your yoni during meetings
- Dance in your kitchen
- Wear clothes that feel sensual
- Eat foods that make you feel alive
- Move in ways that bring pleasure

You're not just changing how you masturbate. You're changing how you live. You're claiming your birthright to pleasure, to aliveness, to your own body's wisdom.

And yes, it's radical. In a world that profits from women's disconnection, choosing connection is revolutionary. In a culture that teaches women to be objects of desire, choosing to be subjects of your own pleasure is subversive.

But mostly? It's coming home. To the body you've always had. To the pleasure that's always been waiting. To the love you've always been.

One touch at a time.

Key Takeaways from This Chapter

- Self-pleasure as spiritual practice offers complete sovereignty over your body and direct access to creative life force
- Mirror work - both genital and full body - heals shame and builds true acceptance
- Creating ritual around self-pleasure transforms it from quick release to sacred practice
- Presence-based practice (vs. fantasy-dependent) deepens your capacity for embodied pleasure
- Tools and toys are allies when used consciously, not replacements for human touch
- Your practice naturally shifts with menstrual cycles and life seasons
- Common challenges like numbness or shame are gateways to deeper healing
- Consistent practice creates ripple effects throughout your entire life

Chapter 6: Yoni Massage for Healing

Your yoni holds memory. Not just mental memory, but cellular memory. Every experience of pleasure, pain, boundary crossing, opening, closing - it's all recorded in your tissues. Most therapeutic bodywork acknowledges that we store emotion and trauma in our muscles and fascia. Yet somehow, we've ignored the most vulnerable, sensitive part of our bodies when it comes to healing touch.

Yoni massage isn't about having better orgasms (though that's often a side effect). It's about coming home to a part of yourself you may have abandoned, numbed out, or learned to endure rather than enjoy. It's about releasing what doesn't serve you and awakening what does. It's about treating your yoni as the sacred, wise part of your body she is.

Anatomy Education with Spiritual Context

Let's get reacquainted with your anatomy - not the simplified version from health class, but the full, complex, miraculous truth of your yoni.

External Anatomy:

Your **vulva** (the external parts) includes:

- **Mons pubis**: The fatty tissue over your pubic bone, rich with nerve endings
- **Outer labia (labia majora)**: Protective lips that swell with arousal
- **Inner labia (labia minora)**: Incredibly sensitive, no two alike

- **Clitoral hood**: Protects your clitoral glans
- **Clitoral glans**: The visible tip of your clitoris
- **Vestibule**: The area containing your vaginal and urethral openings
- **Perineum**: The space between vagina and anus, often ignored but very responsive

Internal Anatomy:

Your **vagina** includes:

- **Vaginal entrance**: Surrounded by the bulbs of your internal clitoris
- **Vaginal canal**: Lined with rugae (ridges) that create different sensations
- **G-spot/G-zone**: 1-3 inches inside on front wall, feels different when aroused
- **A-spot**: Anterior fornix, deeper on front wall
- **Cervix**: The gateway between vagina and womb
- **P-spot**: Posterior fornix, behind the cervix

But anatomy is just the beginning. Each area holds different energy:

- **Clitoris**: Pure pleasure, joy, celebration
- **Vaginal entrance**: Boundaries, choice, opening/closing
- **G-spot**: Emotions, particularly grief and rage
- **Cervix**: Deep feminine wisdom, spiritual connection, profound surrender
- **Perineum**: Grounding, safety, root connection

Understanding this helps you approach yoni massage not as mechanical stimulation but as a conversation with different aspects of yourself.

Step-by-Step Self-Massage Techniques

Before you begin, remember: this is healing work, not performance. There's no right way to feel. You might experience pleasure, numbness, emotion, or nothing at all. All responses are valid information.

Preparation:

1. **Sacred space**: Clean, warm, private
2. **Time**: At least 45-60 minutes without rushing
3. **Supplies**: Natural oil, towels, tissues, water
4. **Empty bladder**: But know emotions might make you feel like peeing
5. **Intention**: Healing, exploration, or simply presence

External Massage Sequence:

1. **Grounding**: Sit comfortably, hands on thighs, breathe deeply
2. **Awakening touch**:
   o Rest one hand on heart, one on yoni
   o Breathe connection between them
   o Hold for 2-3 minutes
3. **Outer massage**:
   o Oil your hands generously
   o Massage mons pubis in circles
   o Include hip creases and inner thighs
   o Work outer labia between thumb and fingers
   o Spend 10-15 minutes here
4. **Inner labia massage**:
   o Gently separate outer labia
   o Stroke inner labia with one finger
   o Try different pressures and speeds
   o Notice changes in color and swelling
5. **Clitoral attention**:
   o Circle around before direct touch
   o Try through the hood first
   o Experiment with pressure

o   Include the legs of clitoris extending down

Internal Massage Sequence:

Only go internal when you feel genuinely open and ready. Your
yoni will tell you - she'll feel warm, swollen, wet, yearning.

1. **Entry ritual**:
   o   Place finger at entrance
   o   Ask permission (really)
   o   Wait for your body's yes
   o   Enter slowly, one knuckle at a time
2. **Entrance work**:
   o   Rest just inside
   o   Gentle circles around entrance
   o   Feel for tight spots
   o   Breathe into your finger
3. **Vaginal mapping**:
   o   Imagine clock face at entrance
   o   Touch each "hour" with same pressure
   o   Notice different sensations
   o   Go slow, stay present
4. **G-zone exploration**:
   o   1-3 inches in on front wall
   o   Feels ridged or spongy
   o   Try come-hither motion
   o   Might feel need to pee - normal
5. **Deep touch** (if comfortable):
   o   Reach toward cervix
   o   Touch gently - it's sensitive
   o   Try different positions to reach
   o   Some need curve of wand/toy
6. **Integration**:
   o   Remove hand slowly
   o   Cup vulva with whole hand
   o   Rest and breathe
   o   Notice whole body

Trauma-Sensitive Approaches

If you're working with sexual trauma (and let's be honest, most women have some degree of sexual wounding), yoni massage requires extra care. Your body might have learned that genital touch equals danger. Respect these protective mechanisms while gently inviting new possibilities.

Signs of trauma response:

- Sudden numbness
- Dissociation (leaving your body)
- Intense emotion
- Muscle armoring (involuntary clenching)
- Flashbacks
- Nausea
- Wanting to stop immediately

Trauma-informed modifications:

1. **Start even slower**: Maybe just holding your vulva for weeks
2. **Stay external longer**: Internal work can wait months or years
3. **Use intermediaries**: Touch through underwear or with gloved hand
4. **Change positions**: Lying on side or sitting up might feel safer
5. **Keep eyes open**: Helps stay present
6. **Work with support**: Consider doing alongside therapy
7. **Honor your pace**: Healing happens in spirals, not lines

Jennifer's experience: "I couldn't touch myself without panicking. My therapist suggested starting by just looking in the mirror. Then holding through underwear. It took six months before I could do internal massage. But when I finally could, I found grief I'd been holding for 20 years. Releasing it changed everything - not just sexually, but in how I moved through the world."

De-armoring Practices

Armoring is chronic tension held in tissue. In your yoni, it might feel like:

- Dense, hard spots
- Areas of numbness
- Sharp pain with pressure
- Involuntary clenching
- Emotional charge when touched

De-armoring is the process of gently releasing this held tension. It's not about forcing - it's about patient presence until the tissue feels safe enough to let go.

Basic de-armoring technique:

1. Find an armored spot (numb, tight, or painful)
2. Apply gentle, steady pressure
3. Breathe into the spot
4. Make sound if it helps
5. Stay present with sensation
6. Notice any emotions arising
7. Continue until you feel a shift
8. Might take 30 seconds or 10 minutes

What might happen:

- Tissue softens
- Emotion releases
- Memory surfaces
- Energy moves
- Nothing (also fine)

Emotional Release and Integration

Your yoni is like an emotional filing cabinet. Different areas hold different feelings:

- **Entrance**: Often holds boundary violations, times you said yes when you meant no
- **G-spot**: Commonly stores grief, abandonment, rage
- **Deep vaginal walls**: May hold ancestral trauma, collective female pain
- **Cervix**: Often contains deepest wounds and biggest breakthroughs

When emotion comes:

1. **Welcome it**: "Hello anger/grief/fear, I see you"
2. **Breathe it**: Deep breaths help emotion move
3. **Sound it**: Moan, cry, growl, scream into pillow
4. **Move it**: Shake, rock, writhe
5. **Complete it**: Let it fully express until it naturally ebbs

Integration is crucial:

- Journal what came up
- Take salt bath
- Walk in nature
- Talk to trusted friend/therapist
- Be extra gentle with yourself
- Know that release creates space for pleasure

Using Crystal Wands and Other Tools

While fingers are perfect tools, some women find wands helpful for:

- Reaching deeper areas
- Maintaining steady pressure

- Energetic properties
- Creating ritual feel

Choosing a wand:

- **Material**: Rose quartz (love), obsidian (shadow work), jade (healing)
- **Size**: Start smaller than you think
- **Shape**: Curved for G-spot, straight for general use
- **Quality**: Smooth, no cracks, body-safe

Using wands safely:

- Always clean before/after
- Warm to body temperature
- More oil than you think
- Go slower than slow
- Listen to your body
- Never force

Working with a Partner

If you choose to share yoni massage with a partner, it requires next-level communication and trust. This is not foreplay - it's healing work.

Prerequisites:

- You've done extensive self-practice
- Deep trust with partner
- Clear agreements about boundaries
- Understanding this isn't about their pleasure
- Commitment to stop anytime

Communication tools:

- **Number system**: 1-10 for pressure

- **Clock positions**: "Touch at 3 o'clock"
- **Yes/no/maybe**: Constant checking in
- **Safe word**: For immediate stop
- **Aftercare plan**: How to integrate

The biggest challenge? Receiving without performing. Notice urges to:

- Make it good for them
- Pretend more pleasure than you feel
- Rush to reciprocate
- Minimize your needs

Rebecca shares: "Having my husband give me therapeutic yoni massage saved our marriage. Not because it was sexy - often it wasn't. But because I finally let him witness my healing. He held space while I raged about past lovers. He stayed present while I sobbed. He celebrated when I finally felt pleasure without pain. It bonded us beyond any regular sex."

Creating a Regular Practice

Yoni massage works best as regular practice, not occasional event. Your tissue responds to consistency.

Suggested rhythm:

Daily (5 minutes): External holding/breathing **Weekly (30-45 minutes)**: Full external massage **Bi-weekly (60-90 minutes)**: Internal work if ready **Monthly (2 hours)**: Deep practice with integration

Track your journey:

- Where you hold tension
- How sensation changes
- What emotions arise

- Which areas awaken
- When you feel most open

The Healing Journey

Women report profound shifts through regular yoni massage:

Physical healing:

- Increased lubrication
- Stronger orgasms
- Less menstrual pain
- Better pelvic floor tone
- Increased sensitivity

Emotional healing:

- Released stored trauma
- Clearer boundaries
- Less sexual shame
- Increased confidence
- Better communication

Spiritual opening:

- Feeling of coming home
- Connection to feminine lineage
- Access to intuition
- Spiritual experiences during practice
- Sense of yoni as oracle

Honoring Your Rhythm

Your yoni has her own rhythm. Sometimes she wants touch, sometimes she doesn't. Sometimes she opens like a flower, sometimes she's locked tight. This isn't failure - it's communication.

Learn her language:

- Swelling means yes
- Dryness might mean not yet
- Pulsing indicates building energy
- Clenching could be protection
- Numbness often covers emotion

The more you listen, the more she speaks. The more you honor her wisdom, the more she shares. This is the ultimate reclamation - not just of pleasure, but of the profound intelligence living in your pelvis.

She's been waiting for you to come home. One conscious touch at a time, you are.

Key Takeaways from This Chapter

- Your yoni holds cellular memory of every sexual experience - healing happens through conscious, loving touch
- Different areas of your yoni correspond to different emotions and energetic qualities
- Yoni massage is therapeutic bodywork requiring patience, presence, and sacred intention
- Trauma-sensitive approaches honor your body's protective mechanisms while inviting gentle opening
- De-armoring releases chronic tension and stored emotion from vaginal tissues
- Emotional release during massage is normal and healthy - integration is essential
- Regular practice creates cumulative healing - consistency matters more than duration
- Your yoni has her own language and rhythm - learning to listen is the ultimate reclamation

Chapter 7: Breast and Heart Connection

Your breasts are not decorative objects. They're not just erogenous zones for someone else's pleasure. They're powerful energy centers directly wired to your heart, your yoni, and your deepest feminine wisdom. Yet most of us relate to our breasts through a haze of judgment - too big, too small, too saggy, too uneven. We armor them in underwire, hide them or display them based on others' comfort, and generally treat them as external appendages rather than integral parts of our sexual-spiritual circuitry.

What if I told you that your breasts are actually gateways? That conscious breast touch can open your heart, awaken your yoni, and circulate healing energy through your entire system? That many women need breast activation to experience full-body orgasms? That your breasts hold the key to receiving love - not just giving it?

Heart-Opening Practices

Let's start with the energetic truth: your breasts are the external expression of your heart chakra. In Traditional Chinese Medicine, the nipples are considered part of the liver meridian, which governs the free flow of emotions. In Tantra, the breasts are seen as positive poles that complement the negative pole of the yoni, creating an electrical circuit of pleasure.

But for most women, the heart-breast connection is blocked. We've learned to protect our hearts by armoring our chests. We hold our breath high and tight. We round our shoulders forward. We literally close off our heart space.

68

Basic Heart-Breast Awakening:

1. **Observation**: Stand before a mirror and notice your posture. Are your shoulders rolled forward? Chest collapsed? This is heart armoring made visible.
2. **Breathing expansion**:
   o Place hands on upper chest
   o Inhale and expand ribs outward
   o Exhale and maintain expansion
   o Practice until this feels natural
3. **Heart opening movement**:
   o Stand with arms at sides
   o Inhale and sweep arms up and back
   o Arch gently, opening chest to sky
   o Exhale and return to center
   o Repeat 10 times with breath
4. **Emotional awareness**:
   o Notice what emotions arise with opening
   o Common: vulnerability, sadness, fear
   o Also common: relief, joy, expansion
   o All responses are information

Catherine discovered: "When I started heart-opening practices, I cried every time. I realized I'd been protecting my heart since my divorce. My breasts had become numb because my heart was closed. As I gently opened, sensation returned to both."

Breast Massage for Energy Circulation

Breast massage is an ancient practice found in Taoist, Tantric, and indigenous traditions worldwide. It's not foreplay - it's healthcare, emotional care, and spiritual practice rolled into one.

Benefits of regular breast massage:

- Increases lymphatic drainage (major detox)
- Balances hormones

- Increases breast awareness (early detection)
- Opens heart chakra
- Awakens sensation
- Connects heart and yoni
- Releases stored emotion
- Cultivates self-love

Basic Breast Massage Sequence:

Preparation:

- Warm room, comfortable position
- Natural oil (coconut, almond, or specialized breast oil)
- 15-30 minutes uninterrupted
- Intention of love and healing

The Practice:

1. **Heart connection:**
   - Both hands on heart center
   - Breathe love into your heart
   - Feel gratitude for your breasts
   - Set intention for healing/awakening
2. **Warming:**
   - Rub hands together vigorously
   - Place warm palms over breasts
   - Just hold for 1-2 minutes
   - Breathe into the warmth
3. **Circular massage:**
   - Start with large circles around entire breast
   - Use full hand, not just fingers
   - Inward circles (up center, down sides) for energy cultivation
   - Outward circles for releasing/detoxing
   - 36 circles each direction
4. **Spiral massage:**
   - Start at outer edge

- Spiral inward toward nipple
- Use medium pressure
- Notice changing textures
- End at nipple, hold gently

5. **Nipple activation**:
   - Roll nipples between thumb and finger
   - Try different pressures
   - Pull gently outward
   - Circle around areola
   - Notice whole-body response

6. **Figure-8 connection**:
   - Use both hands
   - Create figure-8 pattern between breasts
   - This connects left and right sides
   - Balances masculine/feminine

7. **Heart-yoni connection**:
   - One hand on heart/breast
   - Other hand on yoni
   - Breathe energy between them
   - Feel/imagine golden thread connecting
   - This is the key circuit

8. **Integration**:
   - Cup both breasts gently
   - Breathe gratitude
   - Notice whole-body sensation
   - Rest in the aliveness

Connecting Pleasure with Emotional Healing

Here's what nobody tells you: your breasts hold emotion.
Specifically, they hold grief, heartbreak, and unexpressed love.
Think about it - when we're sad, we hold our heart. When we're
protecting ourselves, we cross arms over chest. Your breasts
have been absorbing these protective patterns for years.

During breast massage, you might experience:

- Sudden sadness
- Memories of past lovers
- Grief about aging/changing breasts
- Anger about objectification
- Joy at reclaiming this connection
- Sexual arousal
- Nothing (also normal)

Sarah's story: "During a breast massage, I suddenly remembered being 13 and desperately binding my growing breasts. I'd internalized that they made me a target. As an adult, I'd been unconsciously punishing them - rough touch, no care. When I finally touched them with love, I grieved for that girl who learned to hate her changing body. That release opened pathways I didn't know were closed."

The Positive Pole Principle

In Tantric energy anatomy, your body has positive and negative poles (like a battery):

- Breasts = positive pole (giving/radiating)
- Yoni = negative pole (receiving/drawing in)
- Heart = positive
- Root = negative

For energy to flow freely, both poles need activation. Many women focus solely on genital stimulation, wondering why orgasms feel limited or localized. Without breast/heart activation, you're working with half your circuitry.

Circuitry Practice:

1. Begin with breast massage (activate positive pole)
2. Include yoni touch (activate negative pole)
3. Alternate between them

4. Use breath to connect: inhale up from yoni to heart, exhale down
5. Visualize energy moving in orbit
6. Notice how this amplifies sensation

Results:

- Stronger, fuller orgasms
- Full-body pleasure waves
- Emotional release and integration
- Feeling of completeness
- Heart-centered (not just genital) arousal

Breast Breathing

Your breath can massage your breasts from the inside. This subtle practice builds awareness and circulation.

1. **Basic breast breathing**:
   o Hands cupping breasts
   o Inhale and imagine breath filling breasts
   o Feel them expand from inside
   o Exhale and maintain gentle expansion
   o Creates internal massage
2. **Nipple breathing**:
   o Imagine breathing through nipples
   o Inhale draws energy in through nipples to heart
   o Exhale radiates energy out from heart through nipples
   o Powerful for heart opening
3. **Color breathing**:
   o Assign color to inhale (often pink or green)
   o Breathe color into breasts/heart
   o See/feel color saturating tissue
   o Exhale any gray/dark energy

Healing Breast Shame and Trauma

Most women carry some degree of breast shame or trauma:

- Early development (too soon/too late)
- Comments about size/shape
- Unwanted touch
- Breastfeeding challenges
- Health scares
- Comparison to unrealistic ideals

This shame creates energetic armoring - literal density in the tissue that blocks sensation and energy flow.

Shame Release Practice:

1. Write down every negative message about your breasts
2. Include comments, comparisons, judgments
3. Read the list with compassion for younger you
4. Burn or bury the list ceremonially
5. Speak new truths to your breasts:
   - "You are perfect as you are"
   - "You are sacred"
   - "You deserve gentle touch"
   - "You are wise"

Trauma-Sensitive Breast Work:

If you have breast trauma:

- Start with holding through clothing
- Use very light touch
- Keep sessions short (5-10 minutes)
- Work with visualization before touch
- Consider professional support
- Always honor your pace

Remember: healing happens in layers. What feels impossible today might feel natural in six months.

Daily Breast Care Rituals

Integrating breast awareness into daily life transforms your relationship with your heart center.

Morning activation (2 minutes):

- Upon waking, cup breasts gently
- Circle palms 9 times each direction
- Sets positive tone for day

Shower massage (5 minutes):

- Use shower water for massage
- Vary temperature (cool/warm)
- Soap creates perfect glide
- Include gratitude practice

Evening oil treatment (10 minutes):

- Before bed, massage with oil
- Lavender for calming
- Rose for heart opening
- Include lymphatic drainage

Bra-free time:

- Give breasts freedom daily
- Notice how they move naturally
- Let them breathe
- Reduces lymphatic congestion

Mirror appreciation (30 seconds):

- Daily visual connection
- Speak one appreciation
- Notice without judgment

- Builds positive neural pathways

Partner Breast Massage

If sharing with a partner, breast massage requires different awareness than typical sexual touch.

Guidelines for partners:

1. **This is for her**: Not foreplay for your arousal
2. **Ask permission**: Every time, even in marriage
3. **Start outside-in**: Chest, ribs, around breasts first
4. **Use whole hands**: Not just fingertips on nipples
5. **Go slower**: Then go even slower
6. **Breathe together**: Synchronize your breathing
7. **No goals**: Not trying to arouse or lead somewhere
8. **Hold space**: For whatever emotions arise
9. **Express appreciation**: Verbally honor her breasts
10. **Follow her lead**: She guides pressure, pace, duration

Common challenges:

- Partner gets aroused and rushes
- Woman performs pleasure she doesn't feel
- Old patterns of rough/quick touch
- Inability to receive without reciprocating
- Emotions making partner uncomfortable

Lisa and Mark's breakthrough: "My husband thought breast touch meant grab nipples. I'd endure it to get to 'real' sex. When we learned therapeutic breast massage, everything changed. He'd spend 30 minutes just on my breasts, with no agenda. I'd cry, rage, then melt into pleasure I'd never known. Now I can orgasm from breast touch alone. But more importantly, my heart opened to receiving love in a way it never could before."

The Sacred Power of Breasts

In goddess traditions worldwide, breasts represent:

- Nourishment (physical and spiritual)
- Abundance
- Divine feminine power
- Gateway between worlds
- Seat of compassion

Your breasts are not just tissue. They're antennas for love. They're transformers that convert energy. They're wise counselors that know truth through feeling.

When you honor your breasts as sacred, you:

- Open your capacity to receive
- Heal the heart-sex split
- Activate your full pleasure circuitry
- Reclaim them from cultural objectification
- Step into your full feminine power

This isn't about having perfect breasts. It's about having a sacred relationship with the breasts you have. It's about touching them the way you wish you'd been taught to from the beginning - with reverence, curiosity, and unconditional love.

Your breasts have been waiting for this recognition. Your heart has been longing for this opening. The circuit between them, once consciously connected, becomes a river of life force that nourishes every cell.

Welcome home to your whole self.

Key Takeaways from This Chapter

- Breasts are energy centers directly connected to your heart and yoni, not just erogenous zones

- Heart armoring from emotional protection creates breast numbness and blocks energy flow
- Regular breast massage provides physical health benefits while opening emotional and energetic channels
- Breasts are positive poles that need activation for full-body energy circulation
- Breast shame and trauma create energetic armoring that can be gently released through conscious touch
- Daily breast care rituals transform your relationship with receiving love and pleasure
- Partner breast massage requires different awareness than typical sexual touch - it's healing work
- Honoring breasts as sacred reclaims them from cultural objectification and opens your full feminine power

Chapter 8: Energy Orgasms and Full-Body Pleasure

What if I told you that you could orgasm from breathing alone? From visualizing energy? From someone touching your arm? From dancing? What if everything you've been taught about orgasm - that it requires genital stimulation, that it's a brief peak moment, that some women just can't - is only a tiny fraction of your orgasmic potential?

Welcome to the world of energy orgasms, where pleasure isn't limited to friction and fantasy. Where your whole body becomes an erogenous zone. Where orgasm isn't a destination but an expanded state you can learn to access and sustain. This isn't some mystical promise - it's your birthright as a woman with a body designed for ecstatic states.

Moving Beyond Genital-Focused Pleasure

Let's start with some truth that might ruffle feathers: our culture's obsession with genital-focused sex is relatively new and incredibly limiting. For thousands of years, sacred sexuality traditions understood that sexual energy could be cultivated, circulated, and experienced throughout the entire body. They knew that genital orgasm was just one flavor in a vast buffet of pleasure possibilities.

But we've been conditioned to believe:

- Orgasm requires genital stimulation
- It should follow a predictable arc (arousal → plateau → climax → resolution)
- It lasts a few seconds to maybe a minute
- Some women are just "broken" if this doesn't work

- Men's orgasmic pattern (quick, genital, ejaculatory) is the norm

Here's what's actually true:

- You have erectile tissue throughout your body
- Your entire nervous system can experience orgasmic states
- Orgasms can last minutes or even hours
- There are dozens of different types of orgasms
- Your orgasmic potential is limited only by conditioning, not anatomy

Dr. Beverly Whipple, who helped discover the G-spot, documented women having orgasms from imagery alone in laboratory settings. Dr. Barry Komisaruk's brain imaging studies show that different types of orgasms light up different brain regions - proving they're physiologically distinct experiences (Komisaruk et al., 2004).

So why don't most women know this? Because expanding orgasmic potential requires presence, patience, and practice - none of which our quick-fix culture values. It's easier to sell vibrators than teach energy cultivation. More profitable to pathologize women's bodies than acknowledge our vast capacity.

Breathwork for Energetic Orgasms

Your breath is the most direct path to energy orgasms. Why? Because breath moves energy. Change your breathing pattern, and you change your entire state. This isn't metaphorical - it's measurable in heart rate variability, brainwave patterns, and hormone levels.

The Basic Energy Orgasm Breath:

1. **Preparation**:
   o Lie down in sacred space
   o Knees bent, feet flat
   o Arms relaxed at sides
   o Soft music optional
2. **Building charge**:
   o Begin connected breathing (no pause between inhale/exhale)
   o Breathe through mouth
   o Focus on pelvis filling with breath
   o Add PC muscle squeeze on inhale
   o Release completely on exhale
   o Continue for 5-10 minutes
3. **Moving energy**:
   o When you feel tingling/warmth in pelvis
   o Inhale energy up spine to crown
   o Hold breath at top for 3-5 seconds
   o Exhale down front of body
   o Imagine waterfall of pleasure
   o Rock pelvis gently with breath
4. **Riding waves**:
   o When energy builds, don't contract
   o Breathe it through whole body
   o Make sound - crucial for release
   o Let body move spontaneously
   o Trust the intelligence of energy
5. **Integration**:
   o When waves subside, rest
   o Hands on heart and belly
   o Gentle breathing
   o Notice whole-body aliveness

Common experiences:

- Tingling throughout body
- Waves of pleasure without genital touch
- Emotional release (tears, laughter)

- Spontaneous movements
- Altered consciousness
- Multiple peaks
- Feeling "plugged in" to life force

Emma's first experience: "I thought it was BS until I tried it. After 10 minutes of breathing, my whole body started vibrating. Waves of pleasure rolled through me, way more intense than any genital orgasm. I laughed, cried, saw colors. It lasted 20 minutes. I didn't touch myself once. It revolutionized my understanding of my body."

Full-Body Activation Techniques

Energy orgasms require your whole body to be online and responsive. Most of us have "dead zones" - areas cut off from sensation and energy flow. Awakening these areas expands your orgasmic capacity exponentially.

Body Scanning for Activation:

1. **Map your sensitivity**:
   - Touch each body part with same pressure
   - Rate sensation 1-10
   - Notice patterns of numbness/hypersensitivity
   - Common dead zones: feet, belly, inner arms, throat
2. **Awakening dead zones**:
   - Focus on numb areas
   - Breathe directly into them
   - Use varied touch: scratching, tapping, temperature
   - Make sound while touching
   - Visualize color/light filling area
   - Be patient - can take weeks/months
3. **Connecting zones**:
   - Once areas awaken, connect them

- Stroke from feet to pelvis
- From hands to heart
- From crown to root
- Creating energy pathways

Dance as Activation:

Movement is one of the fastest ways to activate full-body pleasure:

1. **Shake practice:**
   - Stand with feet hip-width
   - Begin shaking whole body
   - Start gentle, build intensity
   - Include every part - even face
   - 5-10 minutes
   - Stop suddenly and feel aliveness
2. **Undulation practice:**
   - Begin with pelvis circles
   - Add spine waves
   - Include chest and head
   - Like seaweed in water
   - Let it become sensual
   - Notice pleasure in movement
3. **Ecstatic dance:**
   - Put on music that moves you
   - Dance with no agenda
   - Include self-touch while dancing
   - Breathe consciously
   - Let sound emerge
   - Dance until you feel electric

Sound and Movement for Expansion

Sound is the secret ingredient most women miss. We've been taught to be quiet during pleasure. But sound moves energy like nothing else. It literally vibrates stuck patterns loose.

Sound practices:

1. **Toning**:
   - Start with "Ahhhh" on exhale
   - Feel vibration in chest
   - Try different vowels: Oh, Oo, Ee
   - Notice where each resonates
   - Combine with self-touch
2. **Sounding emotions**:
   - Growl your anger
   - Moan your pleasure
   - Wail your grief
   - Laugh your joy
   - Let body guide sound
3. **Orgasmic sounds**:
   - Practice pleasure sounds alone
   - Exaggerate at first
   - Notice how sound amplifies sensation
   - Find your authentic expression
   - Let it surprise you

Movement principles:

- Micro-movements often create macro-pleasure
- Stillness after movement heightens awareness
- Spontaneous movement indicates energy moving
- Trust your body's impulses
- Weird is good - means you're breaking patterns

Circulating Sexual Energy for Vitality

Here's the game-changer: sexual energy doesn't have to be released through genital orgasm. You can circulate it through your body for:

- Increased vitality
- Enhanced creativity

- Clearer thinking
- Emotional resilience
- Spiritual connection
- Healing and regeneration

The Microcosmic Orbit (Basic Version):

1. **Build arousal** (through breath, touch, or visualization)
2. **At 70% arousal**, pause stimulation
3. **Contract PC muscles** and hold
4. **Inhale** energy up spine from genitals
5. **Touch tongue** to roof of mouth
6. **Exhale** energy down front channel
7. **Repeat** 9-18 times
8. **Rest** and feel energy distributing

Drawing Energy to Specific Areas:

Need healing somewhere? Draw sexual energy there:

1. **Build arousal** to 50-60%
2. **Breathe energy** to area needing healing
3. **Visualize** golden light filling area
4. **Hold attention** there for 2-3 minutes
5. **Thank** the energy
6. **Ground** with food/water after

Women report healing:

- Chronic pain
- Digestive issues
- Heart conditions
- Depression/anxiety
- Creative blocks
- Menstrual problems

Creating Your Energy Practice

Your energy orgasm practice will be unique. Here's a template:

Beginner (Month 1-2):

- Daily: 5-minute breathing practice
- Weekly: 30-minute full-body activation
- Focus: Learning to feel energy

Intermediate (Month 3-6):

- Daily: 10-minute circulation practice
- Weekly: 45-minute energy orgasm session
- Focus: Sustaining and moving energy

Advanced (Month 6+):

- Daily: Integrated throughout day
- Weekly: 60-90 minute expansion sessions
- Focus: Refining and sharing energy

Common Challenges:

"I don't feel anything"

- Normal at first
- Check for held breath
- Amplify movement and sound
- Work with a teacher
- Consider emotional blocks

"I feel too much"

- Slow down breathing
- Shorter sessions
- More grounding
- Integration time
- Honor your sensitivity

"My partner thinks it's weird"

- Start with solo practice
- Educate about benefits
- Invite without pressure
- Find supportive community
- Trust your path

Types of Energy Orgasms

As you develop sensitivity, you'll discover various flavors:

Breath orgasms: From breathing alone **Sound orgasms**: From toning/singing **Dance orgasms**: From ecstatic movement **Heart orgasms**: Centered in chest **Cervical orgasms**: Deep, emotional, spiritual **Full-body orgasms**: Every cell activated **Thinking off**: From imagery/fantasy alone **Energy transfer**: From partner's energy field **Spontaneous orgasms**: During meditation, yoga **Continuous orgasms**: Sustained orgasmic state

Each type offers different gifts:

- Breath orgasms teach energy mastery
- Heart orgasms heal emotional wounds
- Cervical orgasms connect to spiritual realms
- Full-body orgasms reset your entire system

Integration Into Daily Life

The ultimate goal isn't to have energy orgasms during special practices. It's to live in an orgasmic state - turned on by life itself.

Daily practices:

- Breathe orgasmically while commuting

- Micro-movements at your desk
- Sound in shower/car
- Dance while cooking
- Circulate energy during meetings
- See beauty as foreplay with life

Signs you're living orgasmically:

- Colors seem brighter
- Skin feels more sensitive
- Synchronicities increase
- Creativity flows
- People ask what's different
- Joy becomes baseline
- Challenges feel workable
- Life force radiates

Maria, 52, shares: "I spent decades chasing better genital orgasms. Now I have energy orgasms while gardening, washing dishes, watching sunsets. My body has become a pleasure instrument. I'm literally turned on by being alive. This is what I was seeking all along."

The Revolution

Energy orgasms aren't just personal - they're political. A woman who can generate her own pleasure, who doesn't need anyone or anything external to feel ecstatic, is ungovernable. She can't be controlled through shame. Can't be sold inadequacy. Can't be convinced she's broken.

This is why this knowledge has been suppressed, ridiculed, or relegated to "woo-woo" corners. A world full of orgasmic women is a world transformed.

So as you practice, know that you're not just expanding your own pleasure. You're part of a revolution. You're reclaiming the ecstatic technology of your body. You're modeling for every woman around you that there's so much more available.

Your homework? Put down this book. Lie down. Breathe. Move. Sound. And discover what your body has been waiting to show you.

The only thing between you and energy orgasms is practice and permission. You have both.

Now go shake the universe with your pleasure.

Key Takeaways from This Chapter

- Genital-focused pleasure is just one option in a vast spectrum of orgasmic possibilities
- Energy orgasms are physiologically real, documented by neuroscience research
- Breath is your most direct tool for generating orgasmic states without touch
- Full-body activation through movement and sound exponentially expands pleasure capacity
- Sexual energy can be circulated for healing, creativity, and vitality instead of being depleted
- Different types of energy orgasms offer different gifts and healing opportunities
- The goal is living in an orgasmic state - turned on by life itself
- Energy orgasm mastery is revolutionary - it makes you ungovernable through pleasure sovereignty

Chapter 9: Conscious Communication

The biggest obstacle to sacred sexuality isn't your body, your history, or your partner. It's your inability to speak your truth. To ask for what you want. To say no when you mean no and yes when you mean yes. To navigate the vulnerable terrain of desire without armor. Most of us would rather endure mediocre or even uncomfortable sex than have one honest conversation about our needs.

But here's the thing: sacred sexuality requires radical honesty. Not brutal honesty that wounds, but clear, compassionate truth-telling that creates space for everyone's full expression. You can't have transcendent sex while performing a role. You can't open to cosmic pleasure while managing someone else's ego. You can't heal in silence.

Having the Sacred Sexuality Conversation

So you've been reading this book, doing the practices, feeling the shifts. Now what? How do you bring this to your partnership without triggering every insecurity and defense mechanism in the room?

First, understand what you're up against. When you say "I want to explore sacred sexuality," your partner might hear:

- "Our sex life sucks"
- "You're not enough for me"
- "I want to get weird and spiritual"
- "I've been faking satisfaction"
- "Everything needs to change"

None of that might be true, but fear doesn't deal in truth. It deals in worst-case scenarios.

Opening the Conversation:

Choose your timing wisely. Not:

- Right after sex
- During an argument
- When either is stressed
- In bed
- Casually in passing

Instead:

- Dedicated conversation time
- Neutral location
- Both feeling resourced
- No distractions
- Enough time to go deep

Start with ownership and invitation: "I've been exploring some things about my sexuality that are really exciting me. I'd love to share what I'm learning and see if any of it interests you. Would you be open to that?"

Not: "We need to talk about our sex life" (sounds like trouble) "You should read this book" (sounds like assignment) "I want us to try tantra" (sounds like judgment)

The Initial Share:

Keep it personal and specific:

- What you're discovering about yourself
- How it's benefiting you
- What excites you about possibilities

- Acknowledgment of what's already good
- Invitation without pressure

Example: "I've been learning about breathwork and energy, and it's helping me feel more in my body. I'm discovering I can feel pleasure in new ways. I'd love to explore some of this together, but I also want to honor what already works for us. What do you think?"

Common partner responses and how to work with them:

"This sounds weird/woo-woo" "I get it. It seemed strange to me too at first. Would you be willing to try just one simple breathing exercise with me? If it feels too weird, we stop."

"Our sex life is fine" "I agree! This isn't about fixing anything. It's about exploring what else might be possible. Like we both enjoy dinner, but sometimes it's fun to try a new restaurant."

"I don't have time for complicated practices" "Most of what I'm learning takes no extra time - just bringing more awareness to what we're already doing. Want to start with something super simple?"

"Is this about me not satisfying you?" "This is about me learning more about my own body. What I'm discovering is that I have more capacity for pleasure than I knew. I'd love to explore that WITH you, not instead of you."

Establishing Consent and Boundaries

Consent in sacred sexuality goes way beyond "yes means yes." It's about creating agreements that honor everyone's sovereignty while allowing for growth and exploration.

The Three Pillars of Sacred Consent:

1. **Enthusiastic Agreement**: Not just "okay, fine" but "yes, I'm curious!"
2. **Ongoing Negotiation**: Consent isn't one-time; it's moment by moment
3. **Celebration of Boundaries**: No is as sacred as yes

Creating Your Agreement:

Sit down together and explicitly discuss:

What stays the same:

- Aspects of your sex life you both love
- Frequency that works
- Things that feel sacred already

What you're curious about:

- Specific practices from this book
- Timeline for exploration
- How to integrate slowly

What's off the table:

- Hard boundaries for each person
- Triggers to avoid
- What feels like too much

How to communicate:

- During practice (hand signals, numbers, words)
- After practice (integration talks)
- When things don't go as planned

Sample agreement: "We agree to explore sacred sexuality practices together with curiosity and patience. We'll start with 10 minutes of conscious breathing before our regular lovemaking.

We'll check in during with 'How's this?' and after with 'What did you notice?' Either of us can pause or stop at any time. We'll try this for one month and then reassess."

Creating Ritual Agreements

Beyond general consent, specific ritual agreements create safety for deeper exploration. These are negotiated beforehand and create a container for the experience.

Elements of Ritual Agreement:

Roles: Who's giving? Receiving? Both? **Duration**: How long is this practice? **Activities**: What's included? What's not? **Aftercare**: How will you integrate? **Boundaries**: What stops everything?

Example Ritual Agreement for Yoni Massage:

- Giver: Devoted to receiver's healing
- Receiver: Committed to authentic expression
- Duration: 60 minutes
- Activities: External and internal massage, no goal of orgasm
- Not included: Giver receiving any touch
- Aftercare: 15 minutes holding, then journal separately
- Boundaries: "Pause" slows down, "Stop" ends session

The power of ritual agreements:

- Removes guesswork
- Allows deeper surrender
- Prevents boundary crossing
- Creates sacred container
- Builds trust over time

Jennifer and Tom's story: "We were stuck in a pattern where I'd go along with sex to avoid conflict. Creating ritual agreements changed everything. When we both knew exactly what was happening and for how long, I could actually relax. Tom wasn't wondering if I really wanted to be there. The boundaries created more freedom, not less."

Navigating Different Desires

Reality check: you and your partner probably won't be equally excited about sacred sexuality. One person usually leads, and that's okay. What matters is how you navigate the differences.

Common dynamics:

You're excited, they're skeptical:

- Model the practices solo
- Share benefits without preaching
- Invite without attachment
- Start microscopically small
- Celebrate any openness

You want slow, they want quick:

- Negotiate both experiences
- Take turns leading
- Find bridge practices
- Honor both needs
- Communicate without judgment

You want spiritual, they want physical:

- Remember they're not separate
- Use physical as gateway
- Avoid spiritual jargon
- Focus on felt experience

- Let spirit emerge naturally

Practices for Different Readiness Levels:

If partner is resistant:

- Focus on your solo practice
- Share your glow, not theory
- Offer one simple thing (eye gazing)
- No pressure or timeline
- Trust attraction vs. promotion

If partner is curious but cautious:

- Start with non-sexual practices
- Conscious breathing together
- Massage without genital focus
- Read book together
- Attend workshop together

If partner is enthusiastic:

- Create practice schedule
- Take turns choosing practices
- Find community together
- Support each other's edges
- Celebrate the journey

The Art of Feedback

Learning to give and receive feedback about sex requires ninja-level communication skills. We're all so tender here, so defended, so sure we're broken or not enough.

Giving feedback skillfully:

Use "I" statements: "I notice I need more warm-up" vs. "You always rush" **Be specific**: "I love when you stroke my inner thighs" vs. "Be more sensual" **Appreciate first**: "I loved X, and I'd also enjoy Y" **Suggest, don't demand**: "I'm curious what would happen if..." **Time it well**: Not during or immediately after

Receiving feedback gracefully:

- Breathe before responding
- Say "thank you for telling me"
- Ask clarifying questions
- Don't defend or deflect
- Take time to integrate

Common feedback challenges:

"You're hurting my feelings" Remember: feedback about technique isn't judgment of you as person or lover. It's information about their unique body.

"I feel criticized" Ask: "Can you tell me more about what you need?" Focus on solution, not problem.

"Now I'm self-conscious" Normal! Say: "I might be awkward as I learn this. Is that okay?"

Creating Communication Rituals

Don't leave communication to chance or crisis. Build it into your practice.

Pre-practice check-in:

- How's your body?
- What do you need today?
- Any boundaries to share?

97

- What are you curious about?

During practice:

- Number system (1-10 for pressure)
- Yes/No/Maybe check-ins
- "How's this feeling?"
- Permission to adjust

Post-practice integration:

- What did you notice?
- Any surprises?
- What wants appreciation?
- What wants adjustment?

Weekly relationship ritual:

- Set sacred time
- Share appreciations
- Discuss edges/growth
- Plan explorations
- Connect without agenda

The Power of Vulnerable Sharing

Here's the master key: vulnerability. Not oversharing or emotional dumping, but the courage to reveal your truth even when your voice shakes.

Vulnerable shares that change everything:

- "I've been faking orgasms"
- "I have shame about my desires"
- "I'm scared I'm too much/not enough"
- "I want to feel more connected"
- "I don't know what I like"

When you risk being seen in your truth, you create space for your partner to meet you there. Armor meeting armor creates deadness. Vulnerability meeting vulnerability creates aliveness.

Mark's revelation: "After 15 years of marriage, I finally told my wife that I didn't feel desired, just needed for my function. I'd been hiding behind being the initiator, the strong one. When I shared my longing to be wanted, everything shifted. She had no idea. That conversation opened depths we didn't know existed."

Building Erotic Vocabulary

Part of communication is having words for your experience. Most of us operate with limited erotic vocabulary - clinical terms or porn terminology, neither of which captures the subtlety of sacred sexuality.

Expand your vocabulary:

- Types of touch: feathering, pressing, circling, tapping, holding
- Qualities of sensation: electric, warm, tingling, pulsing, melting
- Energy descriptions: flowing, building, circulating, grounding, expanding
- Emotional flavors: tender, fierce, playful, reverent, wild
- States of arousal: awakening, simmering, peaking, plateauing, integrating

Practice describing sensation: "That feels like warm honey spreading" "I'm sensing electricity in my spine" "My heart feels cracked open" "Energy is spiraling in my belly"

The more precise your language, the better you can guide experiences and share your inner world.

Integration and Evolution

Communication in sacred sexuality isn't a one-time achievement. It's an ongoing practice that deepens with time.

Signs of evolving communication:

- Easier to ask for what you want
- Less triggered by feedback
- More curious than defensive
- Comfortable with not knowing
- Boundaries feel empowering
- Truth comes more quickly
- Silence feels as safe as words

Remember: Every couple has their own communication style. What matters isn't perfection but willingness to keep showing up, keep revealing, keep discovering each other anew.

Sacred sexuality thrives in the soil of truth. Plant your seeds with care, water them with consistency, and watch what grows between you.

Key Takeaways from This Chapter

- Sacred sexuality requires radical honesty - you can't heal or expand while hiding your truth
- Opening conversations needs careful timing and ownership rather than blame or demand
- Consent goes beyond yes/no to enthusiastic agreement, ongoing negotiation, and celebrated boundaries
- Ritual agreements create safe containers for deeper exploration by clarifying roles and boundaries
- Partners rarely have equal enthusiasm - navigate differences with patience and micro-steps
- Feedback requires skill to give and grace to receive - it's information, not judgment
- Regular communication rituals prevent crisis and build intimacy over time

- Vulnerability is the master key - armor meeting armor creates deadness, truth creates aliveness

Chapter 10: Sacred Touch and Presence

Touch is our first language. Before words, before sight, before conscious thought, we knew the world through touch. A baby separated from loving touch fails to thrive, no matter how well fed. Adults deprived of meaningful touch develop depression, anxiety, and illness. Yet somewhere between childhood and adulthood, we learned to ration touch, sexualize it, fear it, or numb out to it entirely.

Sacred touch returns us to touch as prayer, as healing, as communication between souls. It requires us to unlearn everything we think we know about touching and being touched. Because sacred touch isn't about technique - it's about presence. And presence changes everything.

Eye Gazing and Energetic Connection

Before we even get to physical touch, let's talk about the touch that happens through the eyes. In our culture, sustained eye contact is almost taboo. We glance, we look away, we check our phones. To really see and be seen feels too intimate, too vulnerable, too much.

Yet in sacred sexuality traditions, eye gazing is foundational. Why? Because it:

- Synchronizes nervous systems
- Builds energetic connection
- Increases oxytocin (bonding hormone)
- Bypasses mental defenses
- Creates intimacy without words
- Allows authentic seeing

Basic Eye Gazing Practice:

1. **Preparation**:
   - Sit comfortably facing each other
   - Close enough to see clearly
   - Remove glasses if possible
   - Set timer for 5 minutes (build to 10-20)
   - Take three breaths together
2. **The Practice**:
   - Soft gaze into left eye (receptive side)
   - If attention wanders, return gently
   - Notice urges to look away, laugh, speak
   - Breathe through discomfort
   - Allow whatever emotions arise
3. **Common Experiences**:
   - Giggling (nervous system discharge)
   - Tears (heart opening)
   - Seeing face change (perception shifts)
   - Feeling exposed (vulnerability)
   - Deep peace (souls meeting)
   - Sexual arousal (energy building)
4. **Completion**:
   - When timer sounds, close eyes
   - Take three breaths
   - Share one word about experience
   - Hug or hold hands
   - Integrate before moving on

Lisa and David's breakthrough: "We'd been married 12 years but had never really looked at each other. The first time we tried eye gazing, I started sobbing. I realized I'd been hiding from him, performing 'wife' rather than being myself. As we practiced regularly, walls I didn't know existed came down. Now we eye gaze every morning for 2 minutes. It's better than coffee for connection."

Advanced Eye Gazing Variations:

Soul Gazing: See beyond personality to essence **Erotic Gazing**: Build arousal through eyes alone **Healing Gazing**: Send love to partner's wounds **Power Gazing**: Practice holding your center while being seen

Giving and Receiving Touch Meditation

Most touch is transactional - I touch you to get something (arousal, comfort, confirmation). Sacred touch is devotional - I touch you to give presence, to honor your body as sacred, to commune with your essence.

This requires a radical shift from doing to being.

The Giver-Receiver Dynamic:

In conscious touch practice, roles are clear:

- **Giver**: Offers touch with no agenda beyond presence
- **Receiver**: Receives without needing to reciprocate or perform

This clarity creates safety for both:

- Giver isn't wondering if receiver likes it
- Receiver isn't managing giver's needs
- Both can fully inhabit their role

Basic Touch Meditation:

Round 1 - Receiver's Journey (10 minutes):

Receiver:

- Lies down comfortably
- Closes eyes or soft gazes
- Breathes naturally

- Receives without guiding
- Notices without judging
- No need to respond

Giver:

- Begins with hands hovering
- Drops into meditation
- Touches when moved to
- Varies location and quality
- Stays present with sensation
- No goal beyond giving

Round 2 - Switch Roles (10 minutes)

Integration (5 minutes):

- Share experiences
- What did you notice?
- Any surprises?
- Where was presence strongest?

Quality of Sacred Touch:

Sacred touch has different qualities than regular touch:

- **Presence over technique**: Where you are matters more than what you do
- **Listening through hands**: Feeling what wants to happen
- **No agenda**: Not trying to arouse, fix, or achieve
- **Whole hand**: Using palms, not just fingertips
- **Varied rhythm**: Not mechanical or repetitive
- **Breathing together**: Synchronized breath deepens connection

Common challenges:

Giver: "I don't know what to do" Trust your hands. When you drop agenda, intuition emerges.

Receiver: "I feel guilty not reciprocating" Your gift is receiving fully. That serves both of you.

Both: "This feels awkward" Of course! You're rewiring decades of patterning. Awkward is growth.

Full-Body Awakening Massage

Now let's expand touch to the whole body. In our genitally-focused culture, we've forgotten that every inch of skin is an erogenous zone waiting to be awakened.

Mapping Forgotten Zones:

Areas often ignored but highly responsive:

- Scalp and hairline
- Ears and behind ears
- Neck sides and nape
- Inner arms and wrists
- Ribs and sides
- Hip creases
- Behind knees
- Ankles and feet arches

Full-Body Practice Structure:

Preparation (10 minutes):

- Create sacred space
- Receiver bathes/showers
- Giver warms oil
- Both set intention
- Begin with eye gazing

The Journey (45-60 minutes):

1. **Back Body (20 minutes)**:
   - o Start at feet
   - o Long strokes up legs
   - o Attention to glutes/sacrum
   - o Spine work
   - o Shoulders and neck
   - o Scalp massage
2. **Turning Ritual**:
   - o Giver helps receiver turn
   - o Maintain contact throughout
   - o Eye contact when face-up
   - o Breath together
3. **Front Body (20 minutes)**:
   - o Feet and legs again
   - o Belly with permission
   - o Chest/breast with consent
   - o Arms and hands
   - o Face and head
   - o Return to heart
4. **Integration (5-10 minutes)**:
   - o Giver holds heart and belly
   - o Synchronized breathing
   - o No words needed
   - o Slow separation
   - o Share when ready

Keys to Awakening Touch:

Presence: Your attention is the activating force **Variety**: Change pressure, speed, pattern **Surprise**: Don't be predictable **Breath**: Breathe life into your touch **Sound**: Hum or tone while touching **Love**: Touch like you're touching the divine

Rachel's discovery: "I thought my body was numb in places. Turns out those places had never been touched with presence.

When my partner spent 10 minutes just on my ribs - breathing, varying pressure, really being there - I started feeling electric currents. Now my whole torso is an erogenous zone."

Energy Exchange Without Touch

Here's where things get subtle: you can create profound connection and even arousal without any physical touch. Energy exchange is real, palpable, and often more intense than physical contact.

Sensing Energy Fields:

Practice feeling energy:

1. Rub hands together vigorously
2. Slowly separate palms
3. Feel sensation between them
4. Play with distance
5. Notice the "magnetic" feeling

With partner:

1. Stand facing each other
2. Hold hands up, palms facing
3. Slowly approach without touching
4. Stop when you feel energy
5. Play with distance
6. Notice whole body response

Energy Breathing:

1. Sit close, not touching
2. Synchronize breathing
3. Inhale together, gathering energy
4. Exhale toward each other
5. Feel energy building between you

6. Notice arousal without touch

Auric Massage:

1. Receiver lies down
2. Giver hovers hands 2-6 inches above body
3. "Massage" the energy field
4. Notice where field feels different
5. Receiver often feels physical sensation
6. Can be more intense than touch

Mark's experience: "I'm an engineer - this energy stuff sounded like BS. Then my wife 'touched' me without touching, hovering her hands over my body. I felt everything - warmth, tingling, waves of sensation. It was like she was touching me on the inside. Blew my materialist mind wide open."

Creating Sacred Space Together

Sacred touch requires sacred space - not just physical, but energetic. You're creating a temple between you.

Physical Preparation:

- Clean, beautiful space
- Everything needed within reach
- Phones off and away
- Comfortable temperature
- Soft lighting
- Optional: music, candles, flowers

Energetic Preparation:

1. **Cleansing**: Shower separately or together with intention
2. **Transition**: Change clothes or wear something special
3. **Arrival**: Sit together in silence for 2 minutes
4. **Intention**: Each share intention for practice

5. **Invocation**: Call in whatever you consider sacred
6. **Sealing**: Create energetic container through breath/visualization

Maintaining Sacred Space:

- Minimal talking during practice
- No jokes or deflection
- Stay with what's happening
- If triggered, breathe and communicate
- Honor the container you've created

The Art of Presence

Presence is the secret ingredient that transforms ordinary touch into sacred touch. But what is presence, really?

Presence is:

- Full attention in this moment
- No agenda for next moment
- Awareness of sensation
- Open to what is
- Connected to breath
- Rooted in body

Presence is not:

- Thinking about technique
- Planning next move
- Worrying if they like it
- Spacing out
- Performing presence
- Trying to be spiritual

Cultivating Presence:

Before touch:

- 5 minutes solo meditation
- Connect with your body
- Set down the day
- Open to not knowing

During touch:

- Anchor in breath
- Feel through hands
- Notice when mind wanders
- Return to sensation
- Stay curious

After touch:

- Don't rush to speak
- Feel the afterglow
- Notice body sensations
- Integrate slowly

Sarah's revelation: "I realized I'd been touching my husband for 20 years without ever really touching him. I was always thinking about dinner, kids, work. When I learned to bring full presence to touch, he said it felt like I was touching him for the first time. We both cried."

The Neuroscience of Sacred Touch

Let's talk science for a moment. When you touch with presence, you activate specific neural pathways that don't fire during mechanical touch. Research shows that slow, attentive touch activates C-tactile afferents - special nerve fibers that respond to gentle, loving touch and trigger the release of oxytocin, endorphins, and other bonding chemicals (McGlone et al., 2014).

This type of touch:

- Reduces cortisol (stress hormone)
- Increases dopamine and serotonin
- Strengthens immune function
- Improves heart rate variability
- Enhances emotional regulation
- Deepens attachment bonds

In other words, sacred touch isn't just spiritually nourishing - it's physiologically healing.

Overcoming Touch Barriers

Many of us carry touch wounds:

- Being touched without consent
- Touch paired with violence
- Touch as transaction not gift
- Touch deprivation
- Cultural/religious shame

These create armor that sacred touch can gently dissolve.

Working with touch resistance:

1. **Start clothed**: Practice through fabric first
2. **You lead**: Receiver guides where/how
3. **Time limits**: Short sessions build trust
4. **Safe words**: Clear stop/pause signals
5. **Integration**: Talk about what comes up
6. **Professional support**: Consider therapy alongside

Jennifer's healing: "I couldn't let anyone touch me without dissociating after my assault. My partner and I started with him just holding my hand for 5 minutes while I breathed. It took months, but slowly I came back into my body. Sacred touch gave me back what trauma stole."

Touch as Medicine

Indigenous cultures have always known that touch is medicine. Now science confirms what shamans knew: intentional, loving touch can:

- Reduce chronic pain
- Ease depression and anxiety
- Improve sleep
- Boost immune function
- Accelerate healing
- Increase longevity

But here's the key: the consciousness behind the touch matters as much as the touch itself. A clinical massage might relax muscles, but sacred touch heals the soul.

Daily Sacred Touch Practices

Don't save sacred touch for special occasions. Weave it through your daily life:

Morning:

- Wake partner with gentle face caress
- 30-second heart-to-heart hug
- Mindful touch while showering

Throughout day:

- Pause for 20-second hugs
- Touch with presence during passing
- Hand on heart during stress

Evening:

- Foot massage while talking
- Scalp massage before sleep
- Spooning with breath sync

Solo sacred touch:

- Oil your body with devotion
- Massage your own feet
- Hold your heart when emotional
- Touch yourself like a lover would

The Ripple Effect

When you master sacred touch, everything changes:

- Your nervous system regulates more easily
- You feel more embodied
- Intimacy deepens naturally
- Communication improves
- Boundaries clarify
- Pleasure expands
- Love flows more freely

But the real magic? Sacred touch teaches you that you are worthy of reverent attention. That your body is a temple. That presence is the greatest gift you can give or receive.

In a world starved for meaningful touch, choosing to touch and be touched with sacred presence is a radical act. It's saying: I see you. I honor you. You matter. We are more than these roles we play. We are sacred beings having a human experience, and touch is how we remember.

So start tonight. Turn to your partner (or to yourself in the mirror) and touch one small part with total presence. Feel the miracle of skin, of warmth, of life itself. Let that touch be a prayer, a blessing, a coming home.

Because it is. You are. We all are.

Key Takeaways from This Chapter

- Sacred touch is about presence, not technique - it's touching as prayer, healing, and soul communication
- Eye gazing creates profound intimacy by synchronizing nervous systems and bypassing mental defenses
- Clear giver-receiver dynamics allow both people to fully inhabit their roles without performance
- Every inch of skin can become an erogenous zone when touched with presence and awareness
- Energy exchange without physical touch can be more intense than actual contact
- Presence transforms ordinary touch into sacred touch through full attention without agenda
- Sacred touch activates specific neural pathways that promote healing and bonding
- Daily integration of mindful touch creates lasting transformation in relationships and self-connection

Chapter 11: Slow Sex and Mindful Intimacy

We live in the age of fast everything. Fast food, fast fashion, fast internet, and yes, fast sex. We've been conditioned to race toward orgasm like it's the finish line of a sprint, missing the entire journey in our rush to "get there." But what if the whole point isn't to get anywhere? What if sex could be a meditation, a prayer, a three-hour Sunday afternoon of discovering new continents on your lover's body?

Slow sex isn't about moving in slow motion (though sometimes it includes that). It's about presence, savoring, and recognizing that arousal is not a problem to be solved but a state to be explored. It's about treating your body and your partner's body as sacred territory worthy of patient exploration, not a vending machine where you push the right buttons to get your treats.

Moving Beyond Goal-Oriented Sex

Let's be honest about what most of us learned sex should be: foreplay (the appetizer), intercourse (the main course), orgasm (dessert), done. This script is so deeply embedded that we follow it even when it's not working, even when our bodies are screaming for something different.

The goal-oriented model creates so many problems:

- Performance anxiety ("Am I taking too long?")
- Faking pleasure to meet expectations
- Missing subtle sensations while chasing the big ones
- Disconnection from our partner while focused on the finish
- Feeling like failures if orgasm doesn't happen

- Rushing through experiences our bodies want to savor

Here's the thing: goal-oriented sex is a very recent invention. For thousands of years, cultures that honored sexuality as sacred understood that the journey itself was the destination. Orgasm was just one possible scenery along the way, not the sole purpose of the trip.

Rebecca, a 38-year-old teacher, discovered this after years of frustration: "I spent two decades having checkbox sex. Kissing, check. Breasts, check. Oral, check. Intercourse, check. Orgasm... sometimes check, often faked check. When I finally slowed down and dropped the agenda, I discovered I could have waves of pleasure for hours without ever having a traditional orgasm. The pressure to 'achieve' had been blocking my ability to receive."

The Art of Presence in Intimacy

Mindful sex means being fully here, now, in this touch, this breath, this moment of connection. Not thinking about your to-do list, not performing porn moves, not wondering if your stomach looks flat. Just... here.

But presence is harder than it sounds, especially during sex when we're vulnerable, exposed, and often in our heads about everything.

Obstacles to Presence:

- Body shame pulling attention to perceived flaws
- Performance anxiety about doing it "right"
- Intrusive thoughts about daily life
- Comparing to past experiences or partners
- Wondering what they're thinking
- Rushing to match expected timeline

Cultivating Presence:

Breath Anchoring: When you notice your mind wandering, return to breath. Feel your inhale, your partner's exhale. Let breath be the thread that keeps you here.

Sensation Focusing: Pick one sensation and give it full attention. The warmth of skin. The texture of hair. The weight of a hand. When mind drifts, return to that sensation.

Eye Contact: Keep eyes open and connected when possible. Eyes anchor us in the present and with our partner.

Voice and Sound: Describe what you're feeling. "That warmth spreading through my thighs..." Speaking sensation keeps you present to it.

Movement Meditation: Move so slowly you can feel every micro-sensation. Notice how different speeds reveal different pleasures.

Starting Your Slow Sex Practice

You don't need a whole weekend or a tantric workshop to begin. Start with these simple practices:

The Twenty-Minute Make-Out

When did you last kiss for twenty minutes without it leading anywhere? Not as foreplay, but as the main event?

1. Set a timer for twenty minutes
2. Agree to only kiss - no genital touching
3. Explore every possible kiss:
    o Barely touching lips
    o Breathing into each other's mouths
    o Kissing necks, ears, eyelids

- Using different pressures
- Playing with tongues slowly
4. Notice what happens when kissing isn't goal-oriented
5. Feel how arousal builds differently

Most couples discover:

- Kissing is way more erotic than they remembered
- Twenty minutes feels like forever at first
- Arousal spreads through whole body
- Emotional intimacy deepens
- They want to do it again

The One-Touch Meditation

This practice builds erotic patience:

1. Decide who receives first
2. Receiver lies comfortably
3. Giver chooses ONE body part to touch
4. Touch only that part for 10 minutes
5. Explore every possible way to touch it:
   - Different pressures
   - Various speeds
   - Using fingers, palms, breath
   - With oil or without
6. Receiver just receives and breathes
7. No touching anywhere else
8. Switch roles

David and Mark tried this: "My partner spent 10 minutes just on my inner forearm. I thought I'd go crazy with boredom. But after a few minutes, my whole arm became electric. By the end, I was more turned on than from most quickies. It taught me I'd been numbing out to subtle pleasure my whole life."

Positions for Energy Circulation

In slow sex, positions aren't about deep penetration or athletic prowess. They're about creating energy circuits, maintaining connection, and allowing for subtle movement.

Yab Yum (Sitting Position)

This classic tantric position creates a complete energy circuit:

1. Penetrating partner sits cross-legged
2. Receiving partner sits on their lap, wrapping legs around
3. Both spine straight, hearts aligned
4. Arms around each other
5. Foreheads touching or eyes gazing
6. Rock gently or be still
7. Breathe together

Benefits:

- Hearts and genitals aligned
- Equal, facing position
- Allows for stillness
- Energy circulates between partners
- Can maintain for extended time

Scissors Position

Perfect for extended, relaxed connection:

1. Both lie on sides facing same direction
2. Receiving partner's top leg over penetrating partner's hip
3. Gentle penetration from behind/side
4. Hands free to caress
5. Easy to maintain for hours

Benefits:

- No weight on anyone

- Relaxed for both
- Allows subtle movements
- Good for energy cultivation
- Easy to pause and breathe

Modified Missionary for Connection

Transform traditional missionary:

1. Penetrating partner supports weight on forearms
2. Chests touching
3. Receiving partner's legs relaxed, not lifted
4. Minimal thrusting, maximum presence
5. Focus on micro-movements
6. Lots of eye contact

Benefits:

- Full body contact
- Emotional intimacy
- Less goal-oriented
- Hearts connected
- Breath naturally syncs

Extended Pleasure Practices

Now let's talk about making love for hours. Not athletic, pounding-away hours, but conscious, connected, wave-riding hours.

The Three-Hour Window

Block out three hours with no agenda except exploration:

Hour 1: **Arrival and Awakening**

- Create sacred space together

- Eye gazing and breathing
- Massage without genital focus
- Slow building of arousal

Hour 2: **Exploration and Edge Dancing**

- Include genitals but no penetration
- Practice building and circulating energy
- Edge toward orgasm then back off
- Explore what wants to happen

Hour 3: **Integration and Emergence**

- May include penetration or not
- Riding waves of pleasure
- Multiple peaks possible
- Deep rest and integration

Lisa's experience: "We scheduled three hours thinking we'd never fill it. We ended up going four. Without the pressure to perform or achieve, we discovered rhythms we'd never found in 15 years together. I had full-body orgasms from him breathing on my neck. He cried from the heart opening. We felt like we'd taken psychedelics, but it was just presence and time."

Riding Waves vs. Chasing Peaks

In goal-oriented sex, arousal looks like a mountain - climb up, reach peak, slide down, done. In slow sex, arousal looks like ocean waves - rising, cresting, falling, rising again, endlessly.

Wave Riding Practice:

1. Build arousal to 7/10
2. Pause all stimulation
3. Breathe and circulate energy
4. Let arousal drop to 4/10

5. Build again to 8/10
6. Pause and breathe
7. Continue for 30-60 minutes
8. Notice how each wave differs

What you discover:

- Each wave has unique qualities
- Valleys between waves are pleasurable
- Orgasms become optional, not necessary
- Energy builds rather than depletes
- You can ride waves indefinitely

Communication in the Moment

Slow sex requires a new language. Not the pornographic play-by-play or the silent assumption game, but real communication about subtle experiences.

Useful Phrases:

Instead of: "Does that feel good?" Try: "How does that land in your body?"

Instead of: "I'm close" Try: "Energy is building beautifully"

Instead of: "Don't stop" Try: "This rhythm feels perfect"

Instead of: "I can't come" Try: "I'm enjoying these waves"

The Percentage System:

Communicate arousal levels:

- "I'm at 40%" (warming up)
- "Hovering around 70%" (sustainable pleasure)
- "Approaching 90%" (close to orgasm)

- "Let's keep it at 60%" (extend the journey)

The Pause Practice:

Agree that anyone can call "pause" anytime:

- Everything stops
- Both breathe deeply
- Eye contact maintained
- No one asks why
- Resume when both ready

This creates safety to regulate and prevents override patterns.

Dealing with Impatience and Conditioning

Your body has been trained for decades to rush toward orgasm. Slowing down might trigger:

- Frustration
- Boredom
- Anxiety
- Anger
- Feeling like you're "doing it wrong"

This is normal! You're literally rewiring neural pathways.

Working with Impatience:

1. **Name it**: "I notice impatience arising"
2. **Breathe into it**: Don't try to fix, just breathe
3. **Get curious**: Where do you feel it in your body?
4. **Move it**: Shake, sound, express
5. **Return**: Come back to present sensation

Michael's breakthrough: "I thought I'd lose my mind going slow. My body was screaming 'faster, harder!' But I breathed through it, and suddenly broke through to this field of golden pleasure. It was like breaking the sound barrier - all that resistance, then pure flow."

The Biochemistry of Slow

Here's what's happening in your body during slow sex:

- Oxytocin builds gradually (bonding hormone)
- Dopamine stays sustainable (no crash)
- Endorphins accumulate (natural high)
- Cortisol drops (stress reduction)
- Testosterone optimizes (for all genders)
- Serotonin balances (mood regulation)

Fast sex creates a quick spike and crash. Slow sex creates a sustainable altered state that can last hours and linger for days.

Creating Your Slow Sex Practice

Week 1: Agree to slow everything down by 50%. Notice what arises.

Week 2: Try one 20-minute make-out session. No genital touch.

Week 3: Experiment with wave riding. Build and cool three times before allowing orgasm.

Week 4: Schedule a two-hour window. See what wants to emerge.

Month 2: Begin positions for energy circulation. Focus on stillness within connection.

Month 3: Attempt a three-hour session. Let go of all agendas.

Common Concerns

"My partner won't be interested" Start with yourself. Model slowness. Share benefits you experience. Invite without pushing.

"We don't have time" You have time for what you prioritize. Start with 10 extra minutes. Quality over quantity.

"I'll lose my erection/lubrication" This is conditioning. As you practice, your body learns sustainable arousal. Use aids if needed without shame.

"It sounds boring" Boredom is often fear of intimacy in disguise. What are you avoiding by rushing?

The Sacred in the Slow

When you slow down enough, sex becomes prayer. Not prayer to some external deity, but prayer as communion with life force itself. You discover:

- Your body is a temple
- Pleasure is prayer
- Your partner is divine
- This moment is eternity
- Energy is infinite
- Love is the ground of being

This isn't metaphorical. In slow sex, the boundaries between bodies dissolve. Time stops. You touch the infinite through the intimate.

Integration Practices

After slow sex, integration is crucial:

Immediately After:

- Stay connected 5-10 minutes

- Breathe together
- Share one word each
- Gentle separation
- Hydrate

Same Day:

- Journal insights
- Walk in nature
- Eat grounding food
- Early sleep
- No rushing back to normal

Following Days:

- Notice energy shifts
- Practice gratitude
- Move gently
- Honor what opened
- Plan next exploration

The Revolution of Slow

In a culture obsessed with optimization and efficiency, choosing slow sex is revolutionary. It says:

- Presence matters more than performance
- Journey matters more than destination
- Connection matters more than conquest
- Quality matters more than quantity
- Being matters more than doing

When you master slow sex, you master the art of presence itself. And presence is the gateway to everything - deeper love, richer pleasure, authentic connection, spiritual opening.

So tonight, try this: Set a timer for just 5 extra minutes. Whatever you normally do, do it slower. Notice what you've been missing in the rush. Feel what becomes possible when you give time to timelessness.

Your body has been waiting for permission to slow down. Your soul has been longing for presence over performance. Your relationship has been craving depth over habit.

The slow revolution begins with your next touch. Make it count. Make it conscious. Make it sacred.

Time to stop racing through paradise.

Key Takeaways from This Chapter

- Goal-oriented sex creates performance anxiety and misses subtle pleasures available in the journey
- Mindful intimacy requires presence practices: breath anchoring, sensation focus, and eye contact
- Starting practices like 20-minute make-outs and one-touch meditations rewire rushed patterns
- Positions for slow sex prioritize energy circulation and connection over athletic performance
- Wave riding arousal creates sustainable pleasure states versus quick spike-and-crash patterns
- New communication tools help navigate subtle experiences and build safety
- Impatience and frustration are normal when rewiring decades of conditioning
- Slow sex creates sustainable biochemical states that support bonding and extended pleasure

Chapter 12: Partner Yoni Massage

Sharing yoni massage with a partner is like handing them a map to your deepest self. It requires trust that goes beyond typical sexual vulnerability. You're not just sharing your body - you're potentially sharing your tears, your rage, your numbness, your ecstasy, your history written in tissue and memory. This isn't something you do on the third date or because you read about it in a magazine. This is sacred work that demands sacred intention from both people involved.

Most partners, when they first hear about yoni massage, think it's extended foreplay or a fancy way to finger their lover. They imagine it'll be sexy, maybe spiritual, definitely leading to hot sex. What they don't expect is to become a witness to profound healing, to hold space for emotions they didn't know lived in their partner's body, to discover that giving this kind of touch is as transformative as receiving it.

Teaching Your Partner Sacred Touch

Before your partner's hands ever touch your yoni, there's teaching that needs to happen. Not just technical instruction, but a transmission of reverence. Because if they approach your yoni the way they've been taught to approach women's bodies - as something to conquer, please, or perform for - this practice will fail before it begins.

The Pre-Touch Education

Start with a conversation when you're both clothed, comfortable, and have plenty of time. Share:

- What yoni massage means to you
- Why it's different from regular sexual touch
- What you hope to experience
- What fears or concerns you have
- What might come up (emotions, memories, numbness)

Use clear language: "This isn't foreplay. It's therapeutic bodywork that happens to be on my genitals. I might cry. I might get angry. I might feel nothing. I might have intense pleasure. All of it is perfect. Your job is just to be present with whatever happens."

Have them read relevant parts of this book. Watch educational videos together (not porn - actual instructional content). Let them ask questions. Address their concerns:

"What if I do it wrong?" There's no wrong when you're present and responsive. I'll guide you.

"What if you get triggered?" We'll have signals to slow down or stop. Triggering isn't failing - it's information.

"What if I get turned on?" Natural response. But this session is about my healing, not mutual pleasure. Can you hold space for that?

"What if nothing happens?" Nothing is something. We're exploring, not achieving.

The Practice Sessions

Before working with your yoni, have your partner practice presence and therapeutic touch on the rest of your body:

Session 1: Hand Massage (20 minutes)

- Partner massages just your hands

- Practice giving feedback about pressure
- Notice their ability to stay present
- See how they handle detailed guidance

Session 2: Foot Massage (30 minutes)

- More intimate than hands but not sexual
- Practice breathing together
- Work with pressure points
- Notice emotional responses to care

Session 3: Full Body, Non-Sexual (45 minutes)

- Therapeutic massage avoiding breasts/genitals
- Practice clear communication
- Build trust in their touch
- Notice where they rush or check out

Only after these sessions feel good do you move to:

Session 4: External Yoni Massage

- Start with full body massage
- Gradually include vulva
- No internal touch yet
- Process whatever arises

Communication During Practice

Clear communication protocols prevent misunderstandings and create safety:

The Three-Part Check-In:

1. "How's this pressure?" (physical)
2. "What are you noticing?" (sensation)
3. "What do you need?" (adjustment)

Number System:

- 1-3: Too light
- 4-6: Perfect
- 7-8: Bit too much
- 9-10: Stop

Direction Giving:

- "A little to the left"
- "Slower... slower... perfect"
- "Can you hold that spot and just breathe?"
- "More pressure... yes, right there"

Emotional Communication:

- "Emotion is coming up"
- "I need to make sound"
- "Please don't stop what you're doing"
- "Hold still while I breathe through this"

Sarah and James navigated this: "At first, James kept asking 'Is this good? Do you like it?' every 30 seconds. We had to practice him trusting that I'd communicate what I needed. When he finally relaxed into giving without constant validation, everything shifted. He could feel through his hands instead of through his anxiety."

The Sacred Container

Creating the right environment for partner yoni massage is crucial:

Physical Space:

- Clean, warm, private room
- Massage table or bed with towels

- Natural oil within reach
- Tissues and water nearby
- Soft lighting and optional music
- At least 2 hours uninterrupted

Energetic Preparation:

1. **Individual Centering (10 minutes)**
   - Each person meditates separately
   - Connect with individual intention
   - Release the day's energy
2. **Coming Together (10 minutes)**
   - Eye gazing to connect
   - Share intentions aloud
   - Create agreements for session
   - Invoke sacred space however feels right
3. **The Consent Ritual**
   - Receiver states what she's open to
   - Giver confirms understanding
   - Both agree to communication protocols
   - Seal with kiss or hand holding

Integration and Aftercare

What happens after yoni massage is as important as the massage itself. This isn't pizza - you don't just roll over and fall asleep.

Immediate Aftercare (20-30 minutes):

1. **Slow Separation**
   - Giver removes hands very slowly
   - Maintains energetic connection
   - Might cup vulva with whole hand
   - No sudden movements
2. **Physical Comfort**
   - Cover receiver with blanket
   - Offer water or tea

- o Gentle holding if wanted
- o Or space if needed
3. **Silence First**
   - o No immediate processing
   - o Let receiver land
   - o Follow their lead
   - o Stay present
4. **When Ready to Share**
   - o Receiver shares first
   - o Giver listens without fixing
   - o No analysis or interpretation
   - o Just witnessing

Common Aftercare Needs:

- Physical holding
- Alone time
- Walking or movement
- Journaling
- Bath or shower
- Grounding food

The Giver's Experience

We need to talk about what happens for the person giving yoni massage. This isn't a one-way experience. Givers often report:

- Profound sense of honor
- Unexpected emotional responses
- Energetic sensations in their body
- Deepened love and respect
- Sometimes confusion or overwhelm
- Their own healing through giving

Mark shared: "I thought I was just learning better technique. But holding space while my wife released twenty years of sexual shame changed me. I understood in my bones how much women carry. I felt rage at everyone who'd hurt her. I felt honored to witness her healing. I went from thinking I was a good lover to understanding I'd barely scratched the surface of intimacy."

Common Challenges and Solutions

Giver Gets Goal-Oriented

- Trying to produce orgasms or responses
- Solution: Return to presence, breath, following not leading

Receiver Goes Into Performance

- Trying to have the "right" response
- Solution: Name it, breathe, return to authentic expression

Emotional Overwhelm

- Either person flooded by intensity
- Solution: Pause, breathe, ground, continue only when ready

Giver's Arousal

- Natural but can complicate things
- Solution: Acknowledge without acting, stay focused on giving

Time Pressure

- Feeling rushed to finish
- Solution: Only practice when you have ample time

Partner Comparison

- "My ex did it differently"

- Solution: Each partnership is unique, find your way together

The Evolution Process

Your partner yoni massage practice will evolve through stages:

Stage 1: Learning (First 1-3 sessions)

- Awkward, mechanical
- Lots of verbal guidance needed
- Focus on technique
- Nervous laughter common

Stage 2: Relaxing (Sessions 4-10)

- Less verbal direction
- More intuitive touch
- Emotions start arising
- Trust building

Stage 3: Deepening (Sessions 10+)

- Profound energetic connection
- Giver anticipates needs
- Deep healing work possible
- Sacred container strong

Stage 4: Integration (Ongoing)

- Practice becomes natural
- Skills integrate into all touch
- Relationship transformed
- Both people healing

Beyond the Massage Table

The real magic of partner yoni massage isn't what happens during the session - it's how it transforms your entire relationship:

- Communication becomes clearer everywhere
- Non-sexual touch increases
- Emotional intimacy deepens
- Power dynamics shift toward equality
- Both people become more embodied
- Sacred sexuality infuses daily life

Lisa and David discovered: "Learning yoni massage saved our marriage. Not because it improved our sex life - though it did. But because it taught us how to really show up for each other. The level of presence David brings to massaging my yoni, he now brings to listening when I talk. The vulnerability I found receiving, I now bring to asking for what I need. We're different people."

The Sacred Responsibility

If you're reading this as someone who wants to give yoni massage to a partner, understand the sacred responsibility you're taking on. You're not just touching flesh - you're touching someone's deepest wounds and greatest potential. You're being trusted with territory that may have been violated, neglected, or numbed. You're being asked to hold space for whatever lives in those tissues.

This requires you to:

- Do your own healing work
- Examine your motivations
- Release ego investment in outcomes
- Cultivate infinite patience
- Practice exquisite presence
- Honor the privilege

And if you're reading as someone considering receiving, know that you're not obligated to share this practice with anyone. Your yoni, your choice. Always. The right partner will understand that being invited into this practice is a profound gift, not a given.

Creating Your Partnership Practice

Start simple:

Month 1:

- Read and discuss concepts together
- Practice non-sexual massage
- Build communication skills
- Create sacred space together

Month 2:

- Begin external yoni massage
- Focus on presence over technique
- Short sessions (30 minutes)
- Lots of integration time

Month 3:

- Extend sessions if desired
- Add internal massage when ready
- Deepen emotional capacity
- Notice relationship shifts

Ongoing:

- Regular but not rigid practice
- Let it flow with life rhythms
- Keep communication open
- Celebrate the journey

The Ripple Effect

When two people commit to this practice, the healing ripples outward:

- Children feel the increased harmony
- Friends notice the deeper connection
- Other couples ask what's different
- The relationship models possibility
- Both people shine brighter
- Love becomes medicine

This is why partner yoni massage matters beyond the bedroom. It's not just about better sex or even individual healing. It's about two people choosing to meet each other in the most vulnerable spaces with the most exquisite care. It's about creating relationships where both people's full humanity is welcomed. It's about healing the collective wound between masculine and feminine.

In a world where so much touch is unconscious, where so much sex is performance, where so many relationships run on autopilot - choosing to bring this level of presence to intimate touch is revolutionary.

So begin slowly. Begin humbly. Begin with reverence for the territory you're entering. And trust that as you learn to touch and be touched with this quality of presence, you're not just healing each other.

You're healing the world, one conscious touch at a time.

Key Takeaways from This Chapter

- Partner yoni massage requires extensive preparation including education, practice sessions, and clear communication protocols

- Teaching sacred touch starts with non-sexual massage to build presence, trust, and communication skills
- Clear communication systems (numbers, check-ins, emotional cues) create safety for deep healing work
- The giver's experience is profound too - holding space for healing transforms both people
- Integration and aftercare are essential - what happens after is as important as the massage itself
- Common challenges include goal-orientation, performance, and emotional overwhelm - all workable with patience
- The practice evolves through stages from mechanical learning to profound energetic connection
- Benefits extend far beyond the massage table into all aspects of relationship and daily life

Chapter 13: Healing Sexual Trauma

Sexual trauma lives in the body. Not as memory alone, but as cellular intelligence that says: this touch means danger, this sensation means violation, this opening means annihilation. Your body, in its profound wisdom, created these protective responses to help you survive experiences that threatened to destroy you. The tragedy isn't that your body learned to protect itself - it's that long after the danger has passed, these protective patterns remain, blocking you from the pleasure, connection, and aliveness that are your birthright.

If you're reading this chapter, you likely carry some form of sexual wounding. Maybe it was a clear violation - assault, abuse, rape. Maybe it was subtler - coercion, boundary crossing, being sexualized too young. Maybe it was cultural - growing up in a system that taught you your body was shameful, dangerous, or existed for others' consumption. Maybe you can't even name it, but you know something in your sexual self feels broken, numb, or scared.

Here's what I want you to know: You're not broken. Your responses make perfect sense. And healing is possible - not the kind that erases what happened, but the kind that reclaims what was taken.

Gentle Practices for Survivors

The practices in this book might feel like too much if you're carrying significant trauma. That's okay. Actually, it's wise. Your body knows what it can handle. So let's start with practices so gentle they barely register as practices at all.

The Safety Practice

Before any sexual healing can happen, your nervous system needs to know it's safe now. This practice builds that knowing:

1. Find a comfortable position (sitting, lying down, whatever feels secure)
2. Place one hand on your heart, one on your belly
3. Breathe naturally - don't force anything
4. Say internally or aloud: "I am safe in this moment"
5. Notice what happens in your body
6. If you feel unsafe, open your eyes, look around, name 5 things you see
7. Return to breath and hands on body
8. Continue for 2-5 minutes

Do this daily. Not to achieve anything, just to practice safety.

The Boundary Practice

Trauma often involves boundary violation. Rebuilding your sense of where you end and the world begins is foundational:

1. Stand in the middle of a room
2. Extend your arms out
3. Slowly turn in a circle
4. Feel the space around you
5. This is your space
6. Now bring arms closer
7. Find where your energy field feels comfortable
8. Practice sensing this boundary throughout the day

Notice when people enter your energy field. Practice saying (internally at first): "This is my space."

The Choice Practice

Trauma removes choice. Healing returns it:

Throughout your day, notice micro-choices:

- Which foot steps first
- Which hand opens a door
- Which route you walk
- What you eat first

Say internally: "I choose this." Build the muscle of conscious choice in tiny ways.

Working with Triggers and Boundaries

Triggers aren't your enemy - they're your body's alarm system. The goal isn't to eliminate them but to understand and work with them compassionately.

Mapping Your Triggers

Get curious without judgment:

- What kinds of touch feel threatening?
- Which positions make you want to flee?
- What words shut you down?
- Which smells bring body memories?
- What sounds create panic?

Write these down. Not to avoid forever, but to know your territory.

The Trigger Response Plan

When triggered, you need a plan that doesn't rely on thinking (because your prefrontal cortex goes offline):

1. **Stop everything** - Full pause, no questions

2. **Ground yourself** - Feet on floor, name what you see
3. **Breathe** - 4 counts in, 6 counts out
4. **Move** - Shake, walk, change position
5. **Affirm** - "I survived. I am safe now."
6. **Choose** - Continue, pause, or stop completely

Share this plan with any partners. Practice it when not triggered so it's automatic when you are.

Boundary Practice with Touch

Start solo:

1. Touch your own arm
2. Notice when it feels good
3. Notice when it doesn't
4. Practice stopping the moment it doesn't feel good
5. Breathe
6. Try again with different pressure/speed
7. Build the pathway: sensation → awareness → choice

This seems simple but is revolutionary for trauma survivors who learned to override their no.

When to Seek Professional Support

Some trauma is too big to heal alone. You need professional support if:

- You dissociate frequently (leave your body)
- You have panic attacks during any sexual activity
- You can't feel anything below the waist
- You have intrusive flashbacks
- You feel suicidal when triggered
- You use substances to tolerate touch
- Your trauma involved severe abuse

Finding the right support:

- Look for trauma-informed therapists
- Consider somatic approaches (work with the body)
- EMDR can help with specific traumatic memories
- Group therapy can reduce shame
- Specialized sexual trauma therapists exist

You can do therapy alongside these practices. They complement each other.

The Layers of Healing

Sexual trauma healing happens in layers, not lines. You might feel healed then suddenly hit a new edge. This isn't failure - it's deepening.

Layer 1: Safety and Stabilization

- Learning you're safe now
- Basic self-care
- Finding support
- Stopping re-traumatization

Layer 2: Remembrance and Mourning

- Feeling what you couldn't feel then
- Grieving what was lost
- Anger at what was taken
- Sometimes memory recovery

Layer 3: Reconnection

- Reclaiming your body
- Exploring pleasure again
- Building chosen intimacy
- Creating new patterns

You might cycle through these layers many times. Each pass goes deeper.

Rebecca's journey: "I thought I'd dealt with my rape in therapy. Then I started yoni massage and found terror locked in my vaginal walls. I had to go back to safety practices. It felt like failure until my therapist explained I was healing a deeper layer. My mind had healed but my tissues still held the memory."

Somatic Healing Approaches

Talk therapy alone rarely heals sexual trauma because trauma lives in the body. You need body-based (somatic) approaches:

Shaking Practice Animals shake after trauma to discharge the energy. Humans have socialized ourselves out of this natural response:

1. Stand with feet hip-width apart
2. Begin gentle bouncing
3. Let shaking move through your body
4. Include arms, head, making sound
5. 5-10 minutes
6. Stop and stand still
7. Notice the aliveness

Do this whenever you feel frozen or stuck energy.

Pendulation Practice This teaches your nervous system to move between activation and calm:

1. Notice where you feel tension/trauma in your body
2. Find a place that feels neutral or good
3. Gently shift attention between them
4. Spend 30 seconds on each
5. Notice what happens
6. The activated area often softens

This builds resilience and capacity.

Breath for Trauma Many trauma survivors breathe shallowly or hold their breath. This keeps the nervous system in threat mode:

1. Hand on belly
2. Breathe so hand moves
3. Count: 4 in, 6 out (longer exhale calms)
4. If this feels too much, just notice natural breath
5. Practice 5 minutes daily

Breath is medicine you always have access to.

Reclaiming Pleasure After Trauma

The path back to pleasure isn't about "getting over" trauma. It's about expanding your capacity to hold both - the wounds and the wonder.

Start with Non-Sexual Pleasure

- Warm bath with attention to sensation
- Soft fabric on skin
- Gentle self-massage with oil
- Dancing to favorite music
- Eating something delicious slowly

Build pathways that say: my body can feel good things too.

The Reclaiming Practice

When ready (maybe months or years later):

1. Create absolute safety (locked door, phone off)
2. Start with holding your vulva through clothing
3. Just hold with love

4. If emotions come, let them
5. If numbness comes, breathe into it
6. No goal except connection
7. End when body says enough

Each time builds new neural pathways: touch can be safe.

Working with Numbness

Numbness is brilliant protection. Your body learned to "leave" when things got unbearable. Honor this intelligence while gently inviting sensation back:

1. Start with temperature (warm/cool washcloth)
2. Try different textures (silk, fur, rough fabric)
3. Use vibration on surrounding areas
4. Breathe into numb places
5. Talk to them: "I'm here now. It's safe to feel."
6. Be patient - took time to numb, takes time to awaken

Maria discovered: "My whole vulva was numb after childhood abuse. For months I just held her and cried. Then one day I felt a tiny tingle. I sobbed with joy. It took two years to fully feel again, but every sensation that returned felt like coming home."

Integration Strategies

Healing happens between sessions, in how you integrate what arises:

Journaling Prompts:

- What did my body tell me today?
- What protection am I ready to release?
- What pleasure am I ready to receive?
- What choice did I make from empowerment?

148

Movement Integration:

- Dance what you're feeling
- Walk in nature
- Swim (water is deeply healing)
- Yoga or stretching
- Any movement that feels good

Creative Expression:

- Draw your sensations
- Make sounds/music
- Write poetry
- Create altars
- Work with clay

Let your body speak through any medium except words sometimes.

Navigating Relationships

Healing sexual trauma while in relationship adds complexity:

For Survivors:

- You don't owe anyone your healing journey
- You can take breaks from sexual activity
- Your pace is the only pace
- Triggered doesn't mean broken
- You deserve patient, conscious partners

For Partners of Survivors:

- Their trauma isn't about you
- Your needs matter AND their healing comes first
- Education is your responsibility
- Patience is sacred

- Your own therapy might help

Communication Strategies:

- Share your trigger map
- Create clear signals for stop/slow/pause
- Debrief after difficult moments
- Celebrate small victories
- Hold space for messiness

The Spiral Nature of Healing

Healing sexual trauma isn't linear. It spirals:

- You feel better then worse then better
- Old triggers resurface in new ways
- Progress feels like regression sometimes
- Each spiral goes deeper
- Trust the intelligence of the process

What helps:

- Track progress over months, not days
- Celebrate micro-victories
- Have support for hard passages
- Trust your body's wisdom
- Know healing is happening even when invisible

Creating New Imprints

Ultimately, healing sexual trauma means creating enough new positive imprints that they outweigh the traumatic ones. Not erasing the past, but building a present and future where:

- Touch means safety more often than danger
- Pleasure feels like birthright not betrayal
- Your body is home not battlefield

- Intimacy means choice not violation
- You are sovereign in your skin

This takes time. It takes courage. It takes support. And it takes practicing new patterns over and over until your nervous system updates its files: I am safe now. Touch can be good. Pleasure is mine to claim. My body belongs to me.

Every time you choose your boundary, you heal. Every time you feel a spark of pleasure, you heal. Every time you say no OR yes from a place of power, you heal.

You're not just healing yourself. You're healing the collective wound, showing others what's possible, raising children who won't need chapters like this.

Your healing matters. You matter. And no matter what happened to you, your capacity for pleasure, joy, and sacred sexuality remains intact, waiting for you to feel safe enough to reclaim it.

One breath at a time. One choice at a time. One gentle touch at a time.

Welcome home to your body. She's been waiting for you.

Key Takeaways from This Chapter

- Sexual trauma lives in the body as protective cellular intelligence, not just psychological memory
- Healing starts with gentle safety practices - breathing, boundaries, and micro-choices
- Triggers are your body's alarm system; work with them compassionately through grounding and movement
- Professional support is essential for severe trauma - somatic approaches work best
- Healing happens in spiral layers: safety/stabilization, remembrance/mourning, and reconnection

- Body-based practices like shaking, pendulation, and breathwork help discharge trapped trauma
- Numbness is protective; gentle patience and varied stimulation can reawaken sensation
- Creating new positive imprints gradually outweighs traumatic ones without erasing the past

Chapter 14: Sacred Sexuality Through Life Stages

Your sexual energy doesn't exist in a vacuum. It dances with your hormones, shifts with your life experiences, and transforms through every major passage you navigate. Yet most of us received a one-size-fits-all model of sexuality that pretends a 20-year-old body responds the same as a postpartum body, that menopause means the end of good sex, that pregnancy is a sexual wasteland. This thinking robs us of the unique gifts each life stage offers.

The truth? Every phase of your life offers a different doorway into sacred sexuality. Your cycling years teach you rhythm. Pregnancy shows you creation. Postpartum demands integration. Perimenopause invites depth. Menopause initiates you into your crone power. Each transition, when met with consciousness rather than resistance, becomes a spiritual and sexual evolution.

Menstrual Cycle Practices

If you bleed, you have a built-in sacred sexuality practice. Your cycle is a monthly journey through different energetic states, each offering unique access to pleasure, power, and wisdom. But most of us were taught to see our cycles as inconvenient at best, shameful at worst. We pop pills to skip periods, push through with painkillers, and generally treat this profound rhythm as a problem to solve.

What if your cycle is actually your superpower?

Menstrual Phase (Inner Winter) Days 1-5 (approximately)

Your energy turns inward. The veil between worlds thins. Your intuition heightens. This isn't a time to push through - it's a time to receive visions.

Sexual practices for bleeding time:

- Gentle vulva holding with loving presence
- Breast massage to ease cramps
- Visualization practices
- Energy orgasms without genital touch
- Sacred rest as sexual practice

Many women report:

- Heightened sensitivity (can be overwhelming)
- Deep emotional releases
- Profound spiritual experiences
- Need for gentleness
- Aversion to penetration

Honor what your body wants. Some women feel deeply sexual during bleeding, others need complete rest. Both are sacred.

Follicular Phase (Inner Spring) Days 6-13 (approximately)

Energy rises. You feel reborn. Curiosity awakens. Your body prepares for possibility.

Sexual practices for follicular phase:

- Playful exploration
- Trying new techniques
- Increased cardio/movement practices
- Building arousal slowly
- External stimulation focus

What to expect:

- Increasing lubrication
- Growing desire
- More energy for practice
- Optimism about everything
- Easier arousal

This is your "yes" time - use it to explore edges.

Ovulatory Phase (Inner Summer) Days 14-16 (approximately)

Peak life force. Maximum magnetism. Your body broadcasts fertility whether you want babies or not.

Sexual practices for ovulation:

- Extended lovemaking sessions
- Multiple orgasm exploration
- Heart-centered practices
- Partner connection if desired
- Channeling sexual energy into creative projects

You might notice:

- Intense arousal
- Cervix softer and higher
- Increased lubrication
- Desire for deeper penetration
- Feeling irresistible

Lisa tracked her cycle: "I used to wonder why sex felt amazing sometimes and like work other times. Once I started tracking, I realized I was trying to have the same sex all month. Now I plan date nights during ovulation and solo practices during my period. Game changer."

Luteal Phase (Inner Autumn) Days 17-28 (approximately)

Energy begins moving inward. Truth-telling increases. Your body prepares to either grow life or release.

Sexual practices for luteal phase:

- Slower, deeper practices
- Internal massage
- Emotional release work
- De-armoring practices
- Communication practices

Common experiences:

- Decreased patience for BS
- Need for authentic connection
- Breast tenderness
- Variable arousal
- Deep emotional availability

This phase gets demonized as PMS, but it's actually when you're most connected to your truth. Use this for healing work.

Creating a Cycle Practice

1. Track your cycle for 3 months (app or journal)
2. Note sexual desire, energy, emotions daily
3. Plan practices according to phase
4. Honor what each phase needs
5. Share with partners if applicable

Pregnancy and Postpartum

Pregnancy and early motherhood create seismic shifts in sexual energy. Your body performs the ultimate creative act - growing life. Yet our culture often desexualizes pregnant and postpartum bodies, as if creating life somehow disconnects you from the sexual energy that created it.

Sacred Sexuality During Pregnancy

Every trimester offers different gifts:

First Trimester:

- Extreme sensitivity (breast, smell, energy)
- Possible nausea affecting practice
- Deep fatigue requiring gentleness
- Heightened intuition

Practices:

- Energy work without physical touch
- Gentle breast massage
- Visualization
- Partner energy exchange
- Rest as practice

Second Trimester:

- Often increased desire
- More energy available
- Increased blood flow to genitals
- Feeling sensual and powerful

Practices:

- Modified positions for comfort
- Yoni massage adapted for belly
- Heart-genital connection
- Channeling sexual energy to baby
- Celebrating changing body

Third Trimester:

- Physical limitations

- Preparation energy
- Deep opening beginning
- Connection to primal power

Practices:

- Side-lying positions
- External massage only if comfortable
- Nipple stimulation (can trigger labor)
- Breath work for opening
- Surrendering to process

Carmen's experience: "I felt most sexually alive when pregnant. Like my whole body was one erogenous zone. I'd orgasm from my partner kissing my belly. But I also needed him to see me as sexual, not just maternal. Sacred sexuality practices helped us maintain that connection."

Postpartum Realities

After birth, your body needs time. How much depends on:

- Type of birth
- Breastfeeding or not
- Support available
- Sleep deprivation
- Birth trauma
- Hormonal shifts

0-6 Weeks: Healing

- No penetration
- Gentle external touch only if desired
- Focus on healing, not arousal
- Breast care if nursing
- Perineal healing support

6 Weeks-6 Months: Exploration

- Check with healthcare provider
- Start very slowly
- Expect different sensations
- Use lots of lubrication
- Honor exhaustion

6 Months+: Integration

- Discovering your new body
- Working with changed sensations
- Balancing baby needs with sexuality
- Creating new patterns

Common postpartum challenges:

- Vaginal dryness (especially if nursing)
- Decreased desire (normal hormonal)
- Body image struggles
- Touched out feelings
- Leaking breasts during arousal
- Painful penetration
- Exhaustion

Sacred sexuality solutions:

- Lots of organic lubricant
- External practices only
- Energy practices without touch
- Five-minute connections
- Reframe what sex means
- Professional pelvic floor therapy
- Patience and communication

Menopause as Spiritual Initiation

Menopause gets terrible PR. We hear about hot flashes, vaginal dryness, and the end of sexual desire. What we don't hear about is the spiritual initiation, the freedom from monthly cycling, the emergence of crone wisdom, and for many women - the best sex of their lives.

Perimenopause: The Wild Years

The 2-10 years before periods stop completely can feel chaotic:

- Irregular cycles
- Hormonal surges and drops
- Unpredictable emotions
- Changing sexual responses
- Sleep disruption

This chaos is reorganization. Your body is preparing for a new phase of power.

Practices for perimenopause:

- Track what's changing without judgment
- Use more lubricant
- Explore non-genital practices
- Hormone-supporting herbs (with guidance)
- Stress reduction crucial
- Communication about changes

Menopause: The Gateway

When periods stop for 12 months, you've crossed the threshold. What dies: your reproductive capacity. What's born: your crone power.

Physical changes:

- Vaginal tissue thinner

- Less natural lubrication
- Possible decreased libido
- Different orgasmic patterns
- Need for longer arousal

Energetic changes:

- No longer cycling with moon
- Steady energy available
- Decreased people-pleasing
- Increased truth-telling
- Spiritual channels opening

Sacred sexuality practices:

- Daily vaginal massage with oil
- Extended arousal practices
- Heart-centered sexuality
- Energy orgasms
- Cervical awakening
- Jade egg practices

Susan, 58, shares: "Everyone told me menopause would kill my sex life. Instead, it freed it. Without pregnancy fears or monthly bleeding, I could explore continuously. I discovered cervical orgasms at 55. I learned to ejaculate at 57. My partner and I make love for hours. I wish I'd known this was possible."

Working with Changes

Each life stage brings changes that can feel like losses or gains, depending on perspective:

Vaginal changes:

- Use quality lubricant always
- Daily vaginal massage maintains tissue

- Vaginal moisturizers help
- Bioidentical hormones an option
- Patience with arousal

Desire changes:

- Responsive vs spontaneous desire
- Need more warm-up time
- Mental/emotional connection crucial
- Schedule intimacy
- Redefine what desire means

Orgasm changes:

- May take longer
- Different quality
- Need different stimulation
- Multiple orgasms easier
- Energy orgasms more accessible

Body image changes:

- Every stage brings body changes
- Practice mirror work
- Focus on sensation not appearance
- Find beauty in your season
- Celebrate your body's journey

Creating Practice for Your Stage

Your practice needs to honor where you are:

If cycling:

- Monthly practices aligned with phases
- Use cycle as spiritual practice
- Honor the rhythm

If pregnant:

- Gentle adaptation
- Include baby energetically
- Prepare for birth

If postpartum:

- Patience and gentleness
- Micro-practices
- Redefine sexuality

If perimenopausal:

- Track changes with curiosity
- Adapt as needed
- Extra self-care

If menopausal:

- Celebrate the freedom
- Explore new territories
- Claim crone power

The Spiral of Sexual Seasons

Your sexual journey isn't linear - it spirals. Each phase builds on the last while offering new gifts:

- Maiden years: Discovering pleasure
- Mother years: Creating life (literally or figuratively)
- Crone years: Wisdom and freedom

But these aren't rigid categories. You might feel maiden energy at 60 or crone energy at 30. You cycle through all three in different ways throughout life.

What matters is honoring where you are while staying open to evolution. Your 25-year-old sexuality teaches you passion. Your 35-year-old sexuality teaches you depth. Your 45-year-old sexuality teaches you authenticity. Your 55+ sexuality teaches you freedom.

Each stage strips away what's inauthentic and reveals more of your true sexual self. Not despite the changes, but because of them.

Rachel's wisdom: "I'm 68 and having the best sex of my life. Not because my body works like it did at 20, but because I know myself. I've stopped performing. I've claimed my pleasure. I've integrated all the parts of myself. Every wrinkle represents wisdom earned. Every change in my body represents a initiation passed. I wouldn't go back for anything."

Integration Across Stages

No matter your life stage:

1. Honor your body's wisdom
2. Adapt practices to your reality
3. Communicate changes openly
4. Seek support when needed
5. Celebrate your season
6. Trust the journey

Your sexuality is designed to evolve. Fighting that evolution creates suffering. Embracing it creates expansion.

You're not the same sexual being you were ten years ago. Thank goddess. You're becoming more yourself with every passing season. And that self - in all her stages, changes, and transformations - is sacred, sexual, and endlessly creative.

Welcome to your season. It's exactly where you need to be.

Key Takeaways from This Chapter

- Each life stage offers unique doorways into sacred sexuality - none better or worse, all sacred
- Menstrual cycles provide built-in sacred sexuality practice with four distinct energetic phases
- Pregnancy increases sensitivity and life force; each trimester offers different gifts and practices
- Postpartum requires patience and redefinition of sexuality while honoring the profound changes
- Perimenopause chaos is reorganization preparing for new power and freedom
- Menopause initiates crone wisdom and, for many, the best sex of their lives
- Physical changes at every stage can be worked with through adapted practices and perspective
- Your sexuality spirals through maiden, mother, and crone energies throughout life

Chapter 15: Creating Sustainable Practice

Most women approach sacred sexuality like a New Year's resolution. They read the book, feel inspired, practice intensely for two weeks, then life happens. The kids get sick. Work explodes. They're too tired. They forget. Six months later, they're back where they started, wondering why nothing ever really changes.

Here's what nobody tells you: the magic isn't in the peak experiences or the mind-blowing breakthroughs. It's in showing up Tuesday after Tuesday, touching yourself with presence even when you'd rather watch Netflix. It's in the five-minute morning practice that slowly rewires your nervous system. It's in choosing connection over checking out, again and again, until presence becomes your default mode.

Sustainable practice isn't about perfection. It's about creating a relationship with your sexual energy that can weather real life - the exhaustion, the stress, the times when you feel about as sexual as a dishrag. Because that's when you need these practices most.

Daily Energy Cultivation

Your sexual energy isn't separate from your life force energy. When you cultivate one, you enhance the other. This means you can work with your sexual energy throughout your day without anyone knowing you're doing sacred sexuality practice.

The Morning Activation (5 minutes)

Before your feet hit the floor:

1. Place hands on heart and yoni
2. Take 5 deep breaths, imagining breath flowing between these centers
3. Gently squeeze and release pelvic floor muscles 9 times
4. Set an intention for how you want to feel in your body today
5. Stretch like a cat waking up

This simple practice:

- Activates your sexual energy for the day
- Connects heart and sex centers
- Awakens pelvic floor awareness
- Sets embodied intention
- Takes less time than checking Instagram

Micro-Practices Throughout the Day

At red lights: Do kegel pulses with breath. Inhale and squeeze, exhale and release. Nobody knows you're toning your pelvic floor and building sexual energy.

While walking: Feel your hips moving. Let them sway a little more. Breathe into your pelvis. Walking becomes moving meditation.

In the shower: This is your daily self-love ritual. Touch yourself like a lover would. Use nice soap. Make it sensual, not just functional.

While cooking: Dance a little. Stir with your hips. Taste with presence. Cooking is alchemy - pure creative/sexual energy.

Before sleep: Hold your vulva with one hand, heart with the other. Just hold with love. Say "thank you" to your body. Takes 30 seconds.

Maria integrated these practices: "I used to think I needed an hour of tantric breathing to maintain my practice. Now I weave it through everything. My sexual energy stays online because I'm tending it all day in tiny ways. By evening, I'm already warmed up."

Monthly and Seasonal Rituals

While daily practices create consistency, monthly and seasonal rituals create depth. These longer practices are where transformation happens.

Monthly Practice Menu

Choose what calls to you each month:

New Moon Ritual (2 hours)

- Deep yoni massage focusing on release
- Journal what you're ready to let go
- Set intentions for the cycle ahead
- Rest and integrate

Full Moon Ritual (2 hours)

- Celebration practice - what brings you pleasure?
- Dance, self-pleasure, creative expression
- Harvest the month's insights
- Share or create from this energy

Menstrual Ritual (if cycling)

- Day 1-2: Rest and vision
- Create sacred space for bleeding
- Journal dreams and insights
- Honor the death/rebirth cycle

Seasonal Transitions

Spring Equinox: New growth

- What sexual patterns want to bloom?
- Plant seeds through intention
- Practice saying yes to pleasure
- Clear old energy from yoni

Summer Solstice: Full flowering

- Celebrate your sexual power
- Extended pleasure practices
- Share your gifts (teaching, creating)
- Dance, move, express fully

Fall Equinox: Harvest

- What have you learned?
- Practice gratitude for your body
- Begin turning inward
- Release what's complete

Winter Solstice: Deep rest

- Longest night = deepest practice
- Journey into your cave/womb
- Listen for ancient wisdom
- Dream your next becoming

Building Community and Finding Support

Sacred sexuality can feel isolating. You're doing this deep work, having these incredible experiences, and you can't exactly chat about it at the PTA meeting. Finding community changes everything.

Where to Find Your People

Women's circles: Look for red tent gatherings, women's temples, goddess groups. Even if they're not specifically about sexuality, conscious women's circles often welcome these conversations.

Workshops and retreats: Taking a weekend workshop gives you instant community. Look for tantric events, women's sexuality workshops, embodiment retreats.

Online communities: Private Facebook groups, forums, and online courses create connection without geographic limits. Screen carefully for quality and safety.

Create your own: Start a book club with this book. Invite three trusted friends. Meet monthly to discuss practices and experiences.

What to Look For

Healthy communities have:

- Clear boundaries and agreements
- Respect for where everyone is on their journey
- No pressure to share or practice beyond comfort
- Experienced facilitators
- Focus on empowerment, not fixing
- Diversity of ages, bodies, experiences

Red flags:

- Pressure to be sexual with anyone
- Guru worship dynamics
- Expensive pyramid schemes
- Lack of boundaries
- Male leaders without female co-leaders

- Promises of instant transformation

Laura's experience: "I felt like a freak doing these practices alone. Then I found a women's temple in my city. Just being in a room with 20 women openly talking about yoni massage and energy orgasms normalized everything. Now I have sisters who understand this journey."

Your Continuing Journey

Here's something crucial: there is no arriving. No point where you've "mastered" sacred sexuality and you're done. Your sexual energy will keep teaching you until your last breath. And that's the beauty of it.

The Spiral Path

Your journey will spiral through:

Awakening phases: Everything is new! Amazing discoveries! You want to tell everyone! Energy is high, practices feel easy.

Integration phases: The newness wears off. You're integrating changes. Might feel boring. This is where sustainable practice is built.

Deepening phases: Layers you didn't know existed reveal themselves. Often brings up shadow work. Can feel intense or destabilizing.

Plateau phases: Nothing seems to be happening. Old practices stop working. You wonder if you're doing it wrong. (You're not - you're preparing for a leap.)

Quantum leap phases: Sudden breakthrough to new level. Often after a plateau. Everything reorganizes. New capacities come online.

Each spiral goes deeper. What thrilled you last year might feel basic now. That's growth, not failure.

Tracking Your Journey

Keep a practice journal:

- Date and practice done
- Body sensations noticed
- Emotions that arose
- Insights received
- Energy levels before/after
- Cycle day if relevant

Review monthly:

- What patterns do you see?
- What's shifting?
- What wants more attention?
- What can you celebrate?

When Practice Feels Hard

Because it will. You'll hit walls where:

- Everything feels numb
- You're too tired to care
- Old trauma surfaces
- You doubt it's worth it
- Life feels too chaotic

This is when you need practice most, but also when you need to be gentlest with yourself.

Minimum Viable Practice

When you can't do your full practice:

- 30 seconds of conscious breathing
- Touch your heart and say "I love you"
- One minute of hip circles while brushing teeth
- Hold your vulva while falling asleep
- Dance to one song

Something is always better than nothing. The channel stays open with even tiny attention.

Adapting to Life Changes

Your practice will need to shift with:

Relationship changes: New partner, breakup, marriage, divorce - each requires practice adjustment. Don't abandon practice during transitions. That's when you need your center most.

Health challenges: Illness, surgery, chronic conditions - adapt rather than stop. Energy practices work when physical ones don't.

Life transitions: New job, moving, caring for parents, empty nest - each phase needs different support. Let your practice meet you where you are.

Schedule changes: Busy seasons happen. Have minimal practices for crunch times and fuller practices for spacious times.

Rachel's wisdom: "I've maintained a practice for 12 years through divorce, cancer, remarriage, and menopause. The practice itself kept changing, but my commitment to staying connected to my sexual energy never wavered. It's been my North Star through everything."

Integration Strategies

The real work happens between formal practices. Integration is how transformation sticks.

Daily integration:

- Notice how you feel different
- Apply presence to daily activities
- Use your sexual energy for creativity
- Stay connected to your body

Weekly integration:

- Journal about the week's experiences
- Share with a friend or partner
- Create something from your energy
- Adjust practices based on what you learned

Monthly integration:

- Review your journal
- Celebrate growth
- Notice patterns
- Set intentions for next month

The Ripple Effect

As you maintain practice over time, watch for:

Personal changes:

- Increased confidence
- Better boundaries
- More creativity
- Improved health
- Deeper intuition
- Greater joy

Relationship changes:

- Clearer communication
- Deeper intimacy
- Better sex
- Healthier dynamics
- Attracting conscious partners

Life changes:

- Work aligned with purpose
- Friendships that nourish
- Living more authentically
- Magnetizing opportunities
- Trusting life flow

These aren't promises - they're common experiences when you commit to practice.

Creating Your Personal Practice Plan

Design a practice that works for YOUR life:

Daily Minimums (5-10 minutes):

- Choose 1-2 micro-practices
- Same time each day
- Non-negotiable like brushing teeth

Weekly Practices (30-60 minutes):

- Choose one longer practice
- Schedule like an appointment
- Protect this time fiercely

Monthly Rituals (2-3 hours):

- Deep practice or ritual
- Mark on calendar in advance
- Treat as sacred commitment

Quarterly Reviews:

- What's working?
- What needs adjustment?
- What wants to emerge?
- Celebrate progress

Annual Visioning:

- Where has this journey taken you?
- What's next calling?
- How will you deepen?
- What support do you need?

The Long Game

Building a sustainable sacred sexuality practice is playing the long game. You're not trying to fix yourself quickly. You're creating a lifelong relationship with your sexual energy.

This means:

- Progress isn't always linear
- Small consistent actions create big changes
- Patience is as important as passion
- Community sustains individual practice
- Integration matters more than peak experiences
- Your practice will keep evolving
- Trust the process even when you can't see results

After five years of consistent practice, you'll look back amazed at who you've become. After ten years, you won't recognize your old self. After twenty years, you'll be teaching others just by being yourself.

But it all starts with tomorrow morning. Will you put your hands on your body with love? Will you breathe into your pelvis? Will you choose presence over unconsciousness?

The practice is simple. Maintaining it is the advanced work. And you're ready for it.

Your sustainable practice starts with your next breath. Make it conscious. Make it count. Make it the beginning of a lifetime of coming home to yourself.

Key Takeaways from This Chapter

- Sustainable practice is built on small daily actions rather than perfect peak experiences
- Daily micro-practices woven throughout regular activities keep sexual energy online
- Monthly and seasonal rituals create depth and mark important transitions
- Finding community support prevents isolation and accelerates growth
- Your practice will spiral through phases of awakening, integration, deepening, and breakthrough
- Minimum viable practices maintain connection during difficult life periods
- Adaptation to life changes keeps practice relevant and sustainable
- Long-term commitment creates profound transformation that ripples into all life areas

Chapter 16: Living as an Embodied Woman

You've learned the practices. You've touched your body with reverence. You've breathed energy through your circuits and found pleasure in places you didn't know existed. But here's the real question: How do you take this off the massage table and into your life? How do you buy groceries as an embodied woman? Pay bills with your sexual energy online? Attend meetings while connected to your yoni wisdom?

Because that's where the rubber meets the road. It's one thing to feel like a goddess during a two-hour tantric ritual. It's another to maintain that connection while dealing with a screaming toddler, a demanding boss, or a culture that profits from your disconnection. Living as an embodied woman isn't about floating through life in a sensual haze. It's about bringing fierce presence to every moment, staying rooted in your body's wisdom while navigating a world that constantly invites you to leave.

Bringing Sacred Sensuality into Daily Life

The ultimate goal isn't to have great sacred sexuality practices. It's to live a sacred, sensual life. This means infusing ordinary moments with the presence you've cultivated in practice.

Morning Embodiment

How you start your day sets the tone for everything:

Instead of reaching for your phone, reach for your body. Stretch in bed. Feel your skin against the sheets. Notice your breathing.

Even if you only have 30 seconds before chaos descends, use them to arrive in your body.

Conscious Dressing

Getting dressed can be a sensual ritual:

- Feel fabrics against your skin
- Choose clothes that make you feel alive
- Notice how different materials affect your energy
- Dress your body like the temple it is

Sarah discovered: "I used to throw on whatever while mentally planning my day. Now I take two extra minutes to really feel what my body wants to wear. Sounds simple, but starting my day actually inhabiting my skin changes everything."

Sensual Eating

Every meal is an opportunity for presence:

- See the colors on your plate
- Smell before tasting
- Feel texture in your mouth
- Notice how foods land in your body
- Eat what makes you feel vibrant

This isn't about restriction or rules. It's about presence and pleasure. When you eat as an embodied woman, you naturally gravitate toward what nourishes.

Walking Practice

Transform your daily walking into embodiment practice:

- Feel your feet meeting earth
- Let your hips move naturally

- Breathe into your pelvis
- Notice the air on your skin
- Walk like you're making love to the ground

Creativity and Sexual Energy

Your sexual energy and creative energy are the same force. When you cultivate one, you enhance the other. This is why many women experience creative breakthroughs when they begin sacred sexuality practices.

The Creative-Sexual Circuit

Sexual energy flows like this:

- Builds in your yoni/pelvis (first and second chakras)
- Rises through your body
- Can be expressed through:
  - Sexual pleasure
  - Creative projects
  - Life force vitality
  - Spiritual experiences

When you don't express this energy, it stagnates. You feel frustrated, blocked, irritable. When you consciously channel it, you become a creative force of nature.

Channeling Sexual Energy Creatively

After building sexual energy (through practice or daily life), direct it:

1. **Identify your creative outlet**: Writing, painting, dancing, cooking, gardening, business building - anything that makes something from nothing
2. **Build energy consciously**: Through breathwork, movement, or light self-pleasure - stop before release

3. **Direct the energy**: Visualize it flowing from pelvis to hands, voice, or whole body
4. **Create immediately**: While energy is high, go directly to creative work
5. **Let it flow**: Don't think, just let the energy express

Lisa's experience: "I was blocked on my novel for months. Then I started doing energy practices and immediately creating afterwards. Suddenly words flowed. I realized I'd been trying to create from my head. Now I create from my turned-on body."

Your Continuing Journey

As we near the end of this book, let's be clear: this isn't an ending. It's a commencement. You're graduating into a lifetime curriculum of embodied living.

What to Expect Going Forward

Year One: Discovery and awakening

- Everything feels new and exciting
- Big shifts in how you relate to your body
- Possible relationship upheavals
- Creative breakthroughs
- Healing old patterns

Years 2-5: Integration and deepening

- Practices become more natural
- Subtler energies become apparent
- Shadow work emerges
- Relationships transform or end
- New level of self-acceptance

Years 5-10: Embodiment and expression

- Living from your body becomes default
- Teaching others through being
- Creative/professional alignment
- Deeper spiritual opening
- Mentoring others naturally

Beyond: Wisdom and service

- Embodiment is simply who you are
- Natural teacher and guide
- Living in service to life force
- Continual deepening
- Elder wisdom emerging

Challenges You'll Face

The culture will push back: Living as an embodied woman in a disembodied culture creates friction. You'll be "too much" for some people. Good. Your aliveness will trigger others' numbness. Let them have their reactions while you stay in your body.

Old patterns will resurface: Just when you think you've healed something, deeper layers emerge. This isn't failure - it's spiral learning. Each return to old patterns is at a higher level of consciousness.

Isolation phases: Sometimes you'll feel like nobody understands your journey. This is when you most need community, practices, and faith in the process.

Integration challenges: Bridging your practice experiences with daily life takes skill. Be patient with the learning curve.

Staying Connected to Your Body

In a world designed to disconnect you, staying embodied is a radical act. Here's how:

Check in hourly: Set a phone reminder if needed. Ask: Where am I? Am I in my head or body? What do I need right now?

Breath anchors: Use your breath to drop from head to body throughout the day. Three deep breaths changes everything.

Movement breaks: Stand, stretch, shake every hour. Move energy through your system. Even 30 seconds helps.

Pleasure practices: Find small pleasures throughout your day - the sun on your face, a delicious smell, the feeling of soft fabric. Pleasure keeps you embodied.

End-of-day review: Before sleep, scan your body. Thank it for carrying you through the day. Notice what it's telling you.

The Global Shift

You're not just changing your own life. You're part of a global awakening of feminine sexual power. Every woman who reclaims her body contributes to this shift.

Consider what happens when:

- Women stop faking orgasms and start claiming authentic pleasure
- Mothers model embodied presence for their children
- Businesswomen lead from their bodies, not just their heads
- Grandmothers claim their crone wisdom and sexual power
- Young women learn these practices before trauma accumulates

We're literally changing the morphic field of what's possible for women.

Maria, now teaching others: "I started this journey to fix my 'broken' sexuality. What I discovered was a pathway to personal and collective healing. Now I teach my daughter she's sacred. I run my business from my womb wisdom. I've become the ancestor future generations need."

Creating Your Legacy

How will you share what you've learned? You don't need to become a teacher or write a book. Living as an embodied woman is teaching enough. But consider:

For your children: Model body-positive, pleasure-positive living. Teach consent and boundaries. Normalize conversations about bodies and pleasure.

For your community: Be the woman who radiates aliveness. Share resources. Start conversations. Hold space for others' journeys.

For the culture: Challenge systems that profit from disconnection. Support body-positive businesses. Vote for policies that honor women's bodies.

For future generations: Document your journey. Share your story. Be the elder you needed when you were younger.

Integration Practices for Life

As you continue forward:

Daily: Maintain minimal practices that keep you connected. Five minutes daily is better than two hours weekly.

Weekly: Deeper practice or conscious lovemaking. Keep your channel clear and energy flowing.

Monthly: Mark your cycles (lunar or menstrual). Honor the rhythm of expansion and contraction.

Seasonally: Align with nature's cycles. Let your practice shift with the seasons.

Annually: Review and vision. Where have you been? Where are you going?

The Never-Ending Journey

Here's the beautiful truth: you'll never be "done" with this work. Your body will keep teaching you until your last breath. Every age brings new wisdom. Every experience offers new openings. Every challenge invites deeper embodiment.

At 30, you might discover your wild sexual self. At 40, you might heal mother wounds through yoni massage. At 50, you might birth creative projects from your sexual energy. At 60, you might mentor others into their power. At 70, you might become the wise crone the world desperately needs. At 80 and beyond, you might embody the divine feminine in ways that heal collective wounds.

There's no rush. No competition. No perfect way to do this. There's only your way, unfolding in perfect timing.

Your Embodied Life Awaits

So here we are. You've read the book. You've learned the practices. You've possibly cried, raged, felt numb, felt ecstatic, wanted to throw the book across the room, wanted to hug it to your chest. All perfect responses.

Now what?

Now you begin. Or continue. Or deepen. Wherever you are is the right place to be.

Tonight, before you sleep, place your hands on your body - anywhere that calls for touch. Breathe. Say thank you. Thank your body for carrying you this far. Thank your courage for beginning this journey. Thank your future self for who you're becoming.

You are a sacred, sexual, powerful woman living in a culture that fears sacred, sexual, powerful women. Your very existence is a revolution. Your pleasure is medicine the world needs. Your embodiment gives others permission to come home to their bodies too.

This isn't easy work. It's not always blissful. Sometimes it's messy and hard and brings up everything you've been avoiding. But it's real. It's true. It's the path home to who you've always been beneath the conditioning.

Your body has been waiting for you. Your pleasure has been waiting for you. Your power has been waiting for you. The world has been waiting for you - the real you, the embodied you, the turned-on you, the unapologetic you.

So take a breath. Feel your feet on the ground. Notice the aliveness under your skin. And step forward into your embodied life.

The journey of a thousand miles begins with a single step. The journey of embodied womanhood begins with a single breath, taken with presence, in this body, right now.

Welcome home.

Key Takeaways from This Chapter

- Living as an embodied woman means bringing presence and sensuality to ordinary daily activities
- Sexual energy and creative energy are the same force - channeling one enhances the other
- Expect ongoing cycles of discovery, integration, and deepening over years of practice
- Staying embodied in a disembodied culture is a radical act requiring daily commitment
- You're part of a global shift as women reclaim their bodies and sexual power
- Sharing your embodiment through living example creates ripples of healing
- The journey never ends - each life stage offers new depths of embodied wisdom
- Your embodied presence gives others permission to come home to their bodies too

References

1. Urban, H. B. (1999). The extreme Orient: The construction of "tantrism" as a category in the orientalist imagination. *Religion*, 29(2), 123-146.
2. Di Marino, V., & Lepidi, H. (2014). *Anatomic study of the clitoris and the bulbo-clitoral organ.* Springer International Publishing.
3. Georgiadis, J. R., Reinders, A. A., Van der Graaf, F. H., Paans, A. M., & Kortekaas, R. (2007). Brain activation during human male ejaculation revisited. _NeuroReport, 18_(6), 553–557
4. Komisaruk, B. R., & Whipple, B. (2011). Non-genital orgasms. *Sexual and Relationship Therapy*, 26(4), 356-372.
5. Pope, A. (2001). *The wild genie: The healing power of menstruation.* Sally Milner Publishing.
6. Mehling, W. E., Acree, M., Stewart, A., Silas, J., & Jones, A. (2018). The Multidimensional Assessment of Interoceptive Awareness, Version 2 (MAIA-2). *PLoS One*, 13(12), e0208034.
7. Kaestle, C. E., & Allen, K. R. (2011). The role of masturbation in healthy sexual development: Perceptions of young adults. *Archives of Sexual Behavior*, 40(5), 983-994.
8. Komisaruk, B. R., Whipple, B., Crawford, A., Grimes, S., Liu, W. C., Kalnin, A., & Mosier, K. (2004). Brain activation during vaginocervical self-stimulation and orgasm in women with complete spinal cord injury: fMRI evidence of mediation by the vagus nerves. *Brain Research*, 1024(1-2), 77-88.
9. McGlone, F., Wessberg, J., & Olausson, H. (2014). Discriminative and affective touch: sensing and feeling. *Neuron*, 82(4), 737-755.

10. van der Kolk, B. A. (2014). *The body keeps the score: Brain, mind, and body in the healing of trauma*. Viking Press.

11. Levine, P. A. (2010). *In an unspoken voice: How the body releases trauma and restores goodness*. North Atlantic Books.

12. Ogden, P., Minton, K., & Pain, C. (2006). *Trauma and the body: A sensorimotor approach to psychotherapy*. W. W. Norton & Company.

13. Mate, G. (2003). *When the body says no: The cost of hidden stress*. Knopf Canada.

14. Porges, S. W. (2011). *The polyvagal theory: Neurophysiological foundations of emotions, attachment, communication, and self-regulation*. W. W. Norton & Company.

15. Scurlock-Durana, S. (2017). Reclaiming Your Body: Healing from Trauma and Awakening to Your Body's Wisdom. New World Library

16. Northrup, C. (2020). *Women's bodies, women's wisdom: Creating physical and emotional health and healing*. Bantam Books.

17. Ensler, E. (2013). *In the body of the world: A memoir of cancer and connection*. Metropolitan Books.

18. Thomashauer, R. (2016). *Pussy: A reclamation*. Hay House Inc.

19. Winston, S. (2010). *Women's anatomy of arousal: Secret maps to buried pleasure*. Mango Garden Press.